A Theoretical Approach to the Preselection
of Carcinogens and Chemical Carcinogenesis

A Theoretical Approach to the Preselection of Carcinogens and Chemical Carcinogenesis

Veljko Veljković

"Boris Kidrič" Institute for Nuclear Sciences
Beograd, Yugoslavia

GORDON AND BREACH SCIENCE PUBLISHERS

New York   London   Paris

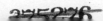

Copyright ©1980 by Gordon and Breach, Science Publishers, Inc.

Gordon and Breach, Science Publishers, Inc.
One Park Avenue
New York, NY10016

Gordon and Breach Science Publishers Ltd.
42 William IV Street
London WC2N 4DF

Gordon & Breach
7–9 rue Emile Dubois
F-75014 Paris

Library of Congress Cataloging in Publication Data

Veljković, Veljko.
    A theoretical approach to the preselection of carcinogens and chemical carcinogenesis.

    Translated from the Serbo-Croatian (Roman)
    Includes bibliographical references and index.
    1. Carcinogens.   2. Valence (Theoretical
chemistry)   3. Carcinogenesis. I. Title.
RC268.6.V4413   616.99'4071   80-2744
ISBN 0-677-05490-4

To Branislava, Nevena, Tatjana and Milena

Acknowledgments

I would like to thank my colleagues, Dr. Dragutin Lalović and Dr. Vladimir Ajdačić, who collaborated with me on the research which eventually led to this book.

Special thanks are due to Dr. Peter Gascoyne of the National Foundation for Cancer Research, in Woods Hole, for his reading of and subsequent invaluable suggestions concerning the manuscript.

And finally, my thanks to Mr. Jay Strouch for his fine English translation.

Contents

A*

Introduction

In the practical use of organic chemical compounds, man has realized an ancient wish : to cease being dependent upon nature. Long ago he ceased to be content with the possibilities which nature has shared through its offerings, turning more and more to chemical compounds which he can himself synthesize. Thus, various synthetic products have appeared, without which the life of modern man could not be imagined; among these are different medications, pesticides, insecticides, plastics, etc, the list is almost endless.

Unfortunately, however, while developing the synthetic processes for new chemical compounds and making practical use of them, little attention has been paid to nature and the laws which govern the living world. Nature has reacted to the ubiquitous presence of pollution, man-made changes to the ecological environment of living beings and other changes in biological processes: mankind has begun to pay a very high price indeed.

One of nature's reactions which is greatly affecting mankind is the incidence of cancer. It has been established that 80–90% of cases of cancer today are caused by elements of chemical origin.[1]

Great scientific and economic resources have been engaged worldwide to try to conquer this dangerous phenomenon. Unfortunately, though, the results obtained are not even in close proportion to the efforts and means engaged. Since after a long period of time satisfactory results have not been achieved on the therapeutic level, a changeover has been made to the development of preventative protection. Primarily this includes the detection and removal of carcinogenic chemical elements from the environment.

However, it has become evident that this task is not in the least easy, frustrated as it is by a number of difficulties. Two basic problems present themselves: (1) the tremendously high cost of these tests, and (2) their lengthy duration (we refer to the most reliable tests performed on mammals). As a result, the number of newly synthesized chemical compounds ready to be marketed each year greatly exceeds the experimental facilities available to test their safety.

Research up to now, which is being conducted in scientific institutions throughout the world, has shown that the problem of carcinogenesis is extremely complex and requires a wide, multidisciplinary approach if it is to be solved.

In this book we will try to analyse the problem of chemical carcinogenesis from the standpoint of some physical principles which directly influence intermolecular processes and, by extension, processes in living matter. Based

1

upon this assumption, we will make use of the electron–ion interaction potential as a starting point. We have chosen this characteristic assuming that the strength of the electromagnetic field surrounding a molecule can provide us with a first indication of its ability to take part in biochemical processes. It seems to us that the structural characteristics of molecules, to which the greatest attention is being directed today, are not sufficient to define their biological activities. For example, it seems hardly possible that transport RNA investigates the topology of every molecule in its midst until the sought-for amino acid is obtained; it is more likely that there exists some sort of pre-selection in accordance with the strength of the molecular field which lessens the number of possibilities and therefore speeds up the process of selection.

On the contemporary level of molecular physics and the physics of condensed matter, an exact treatment of the problem of interactions between molecules in complex biological systems is practically impossible. We shall therefore use the phenomenological approach to connect the microscopic characteristics of organic molecules with the macroscopic manifestations of their performance.

The subject matter of this book can be roughly divided into a group of phenomenological facts which can be easily checked, and into conclusions derived from those facts which may lend themselves to speculation. It is hoped that these results, no matter how many unanswered questions are left, will give new insights not only into the process of carcinogenesis but also into a number of other biological processes occurring in living matter.

CHAPTER 1

The Electron–Ion Interaction Potential of Organic Molecules and their Carcinogenic Properties

We are today witnessing great progress in biological research, especially in the fields of genetics, molecular biology and biochemistry. This results in large quantities of experimental data with which current theoretical research is incapable of keeping pace. Hence we are faced with a situation characterized by theory lagging significantly behind the experimental work that is being carried out, with the result that little is known about the mechanism of certain biological processes. This lack of theoretical knowledge makes the results of some biological experiments, for example, in the field of genetic engineering, unforeseeable and sometimes even dangerous.

The same result is evident in another highly topical, albeit narrower, field of research, that of carcinogenesis. This complex biological phenomenon is at present attracting the attention of researchers working in different disciplines of science; a fact which has provoked a multidisciplinary approach to its study. The involvement of extensive research and material potentials on the one hand, and the lack of a predominant common direction for research to provide guidance for the various efforts on the other, have resulted in a large quantity of divergent experimental data. Some of the findings are pragmatically highly significant but nonetheless have yet to provide an understanding of the main elements of the mechanisms involved in carcinogenesis. This is because theory is lagging behind experimental activity and this may be observed particularly in the study of the phenomenon of carcinogenesis at the submicroscopic level of intermolecular interactions.

There are several reasons for this situation but only two, which in our opinion are the most serious, will be mentioned here. Firstly, the biochemical processes which lead to the development of cancer of a cell are still not known, and secondly the molecular systems participating in this process are remarkably complex. Present-day molecular physics and quantum chemistry have not yet reached a sophisticated enough level of development to allow an exact or indeed even a sufficient treatment of the properties and behaviour of complex biological systems. Consequently a semi-phenomenological approach is the only possible method for attacking the problem of carcinogenesis today. This presumes establishing a basic relationship between a purely theoretical molecular parameter and a measurable macroscopic characteristic. The correlation between two quantities of this kind could subsequently serve as the basis for formulating a corresponding theory. However, the choice of microscopic parameter and related macroscopic characteristic for a given process presents a challenge of considerable magnitude in itself.

When embarking upon this task, various possibilities were analysed and it was decided that it would be best first to study the relationship between the most elementary microscopic parameter available and the most obvious macroscopic characteristic of a given process. Selection of the microscopic parameter turned out to be the easier part of the task. We started from the well-known fact from the theory of condensed matter,[†] that all phenomena are basically dependent upon the characteristics of the electron–ion interaction potential. This led to the assumption that in biological processes too (including those processes involved in carcinogenesis), this physical interaction plays an important role.

The question of which participants in the process of carcinogenesis should be considered important remained open. We chose to rely upon experimental data. According to the World Health Organization, whose conclusions are based upon voluminous statistics, eighty to ninety percent of all cancer diseases are caused by chemical agents found in the human environment. This means that the cancerization of a single cell is due to the direct or indirect interaction between the molecules of a chemical carcinogen with its genetic apparatus. This led us to the use of the electron–ion interaction potential in studying the behaviour of chemical carcinogens. At the same time, we thereby resolved the problem of choosing the corresponding macroscopic characteristic. It was decided that an investigation into the relationship between the electron–ion interaction potential of chemical agents and their cancer-causing properties was called for.

We will not dwell at length on the characteristics of the biological data used in this analysis. Detailed information about them will be presented in the next chapter. As the major source of information about the carcinogenic activity of organic agents, we used the series of monographs published by the International Agency for Research on Cancer, in Lyon.[2] Their results are based upon a study of the carcinogenic effects of chemical compounds in various mammalian systems.

Before explaining the method used to determine the electron–ion interaction potential for organic molecules, we would like to make one clarification. Our approach represents an approximation which no doubt has many shortcomings. Nevertheless we wish to remind our readers that our goal was not to

---

† For those readers not familiar with the details of the theory of condensed matter, we recommend Refs. 63–65.

undertake an exact treatment of the phenomenon of chemical carcinogenesis at the submicroscopic level, but rather to do what was possible given currently available information: that is to find the rôle which some elementary physical characteristics might play in this complex biological process.

Now, in the next chapter, let us describe the major features of the electron–ion interaction and the method of potential calculation, since this potential will be needed in our later analysis.

CHAPTER 2

The Electron–Ion Interaction Potential

The electron–ion interaction potential presented here is deduced from the theory of metals. We shall now offer a brief description of the method by which it was determined, so that the reader can understand its physical basis.

Let us consider the main characteristics of the metallic state — the crystal lattice formed by regularly distributed metal ions in space. The basic feature of this distribution is the translatory symmetry. The space between ions is filled with free electrons resulting from the collectivization of valence electrons of all atoms present. The main characteristic of these electrons is that they do not belong to a specific ion but are moving almost freely through the entire metal lattice. The potential in which these electrons are moving can be expressed within the framework of the diffractory model in the following manner:

$$\langle \mathbf{k} + \mathbf{q} | W | \mathbf{k} \rangle = S(q) \langle \mathbf{k} + \mathbf{q} | \omega | \mathbf{k} \rangle. \tag{1}$$

The square of the matrix element represents the probability that the given electron having momentum $\mathbf{k}$ after interaction with the lattice will change its momentum by $\mathbf{q}$. The set of matrix elements, with respect to all values of the change of momentum $\mathbf{q}$, describes the interaction between the conductive electron and the lattice potential. The value $S(q)$ in Eq. (1) is the structural factor, $i.e.$, the potential component which is exclusively dependent upon the ion distribution in the crystal lattice of the metal. The value $\langle \mathbf{k} + \mathbf{q} | \omega | \mathbf{k} \rangle$ is called the potential form-factor. It describes the interaction between the conductive electron and an ion in the crystal lattice. In other words, the form-factor contains specific atomic-type properties forming the lattice and therefore constitutes the most important characteristic of metals.

Now let us focus on this quantity. The form-factor may be represented by

$$\langle \mathbf{k} + \mathbf{q} | \omega | \mathbf{k} \rangle = \frac{\langle \mathbf{k} + \mathbf{q} | \omega^0 | \mathbf{k} \rangle}{\varepsilon(q)} \tag{2}$$

where the $\langle \mathbf{k} + \mathbf{q} | \omega | \mathbf{k} \rangle$ component is the free ion-potential and $\varepsilon(q)$ the dielectric function describing the screening of the previous component with the gas of free electrons. A structure such as the form-factor of the electron–ion interaction potential in metals is of special importance to us, for if we know this potential for the metal and exclude the component describing the effect of

6

free electrons, we can obtain the potential of the free ion–electron interaction.

The electron–ion interaction potential in metals is, by nature, an extremely complex physical quantity. In the quasi-local approximation it can be calculated for some simple metals on the basis of first principles. In that particular case the form-factor is as follows:

$$\langle \mathbf{k}+\mathbf{q}|\omega|\mathbf{k}\rangle = \frac{V_q^a + V_q^b + V_q^c + V_q^d + V_q^f}{\varepsilon(q)}. \tag{3}$$

Components V_q^a and V_q^b represent the potential of valence charge and the electroneutral complex, given together as

$$V_q^a + V_q^b = \frac{8\pi}{\Omega_0 q^2}|-Z - n(0) + n(q)| \tag{4}$$

where Z is the number of valence electrons per atom, $n(0)$ and $n(q)$ Furrie components of the density of electrons in the closed shell, and Ω_0 the atomic volume.

V_q^c is the potential of the exchange interaction between conductive electrons and electrons of closed atomic shells which, in Slater's approximation, is represented by the following:

$$V_q^c = \frac{1.2707}{q} \cdot \frac{4\pi}{\Omega_0} \int \sin qR |RU(R)|^{1/3} dR \tag{5}$$

where $U(r)$ is tabulated on the basis of Hartree–Fock's functions.

Component V_q^d is the potential of the orthogonalizing hole, expressed as follows:

$$V_q^d = \left[\frac{8\pi Z}{\Omega_0 q} \cdot \frac{n(q)}{n(0)} \left(\frac{Z'}{Z} \right) - 1 \right] \tag{6}$$

where Z' is the so-called effective valence.

The last member in Eq. (3) is of a repulsive nature and is not sufficiently theoretically grounded:

$$V_q^f = \frac{8\pi Z}{\Omega_0 q^2} \sum_{n,l} (2l+1)\langle k+q|nl0\rangle\langle k|nl0\rangle P_l(\cos\theta) \tag{7}$$

where n and l are relevant quantum numbers.

As has already been mentioned, $\varepsilon(q)$ is the dielectric function describing the screening effect by free electrons which are between the observed electron and the ion with which it is interacting. Depending upon the corrections used, different dielectric functions are applied today. Here we will present one of the simplest forms of them and we will use it in our further calculations. It is the Hartree dielectric function, whose form is as follows:

$$\varepsilon(q) = 1 + \frac{me^2}{2\pi k_F \hbar^2 \eta^2} \left(\frac{1-\eta}{2\eta} \ln \left| \frac{1+\eta}{1-\eta} \right| + 1 \right) \qquad (8)$$

where m is the electron mass, e the electron charge, k_F the electron momentum on Fermi's sphere, and η represents $q/2k_F$.

As the above form-factor demonstrates, its computation is extremely complicated, particularly in the case of atoms of heavier metals with a more complex electronic structure. In such cases, when this potential is determined in the above-described manner its accuracy is rather questionable because of the indispensable approximations which must be made in the calculation.

Present-day practice only makes use of phenomenological pseudopotentials. In their formulation the first principles are used as the starting point, to be followed at a certain point by an approximate form, including two or more free parameters. In order to apply this potential we must first determine the numerical values of these free parameters for each given system. This can be accomplished by adjusting parameters to some experimental values which could also be calculated by the help of this potential. More often this is performed with the use of the phonon spectrum, the law of dispersion for free electrons, or the electrical resistance. A whole range of such model pseudo-potentials is presently used.[3-5] We will deal with one of them, since it has some specific characteristics. It is the pseudopotential of Heine and Abarenkov.[6]

This model pseudopotential has the following form:

$$V_{HA}(R) = \begin{cases} -\Sigma A_l(E)P_l & \text{for } R < R_M \\ -Ze/R & \text{for } R > R_M \end{cases} \qquad (9)$$

where P_l is the projection operator which separates from the wave function the components with the azymuthal quantum number l, and E is the energy of the state we are concerned with. Within the sphere which has a diameter of R_M this potential is constant, whereas outside this region it is characterized by a simple Coulomb nature.

Using this potential, Animalu and Heine[7] calculated the form-factor values for all simple metals. As a source of information concerning the state of bound electrons, they used spectroscopic data; to a certain degree, therefore, this potential is of an experimental nature. Later Animalu[8] introduced certain modifications and made similar calculations for transition metals.

The disadvantage of the Heine–Abarenkov potential lies in its complicated

TABLE 1
Values of model parameters β_1 and β_2.

Metals	β_1,Ry	β_2
Li	−0.297	0.585
Na	−0.258	0.561
K	−0.203	0.579
Rb	−0.229	0.480
Cs	−0.230	0.436
Be	−0.961	0.734
Mg	−0.537	0.651
Ca	−0.328	0.698
Ba	−0.227	0.791
Zn	−0.696	0.606
Cd	−0.624	0.588
Hg	−0.641	0.541
Al	−0.790	0.726
Ga	−0.682	0.621
Tl	−0.692	0.576
Si	−0.927	0.661
Ge	−0.866	0.652
Sn	−0.768	0.653
Pb	−0.777	0.598
Sb	−0.833	0.646
Bi	−0.799	0.606
Se	−0.998	0.631
Te	−0.873	0.647

analytical form. In their efforts to overcome the above-mentioned difficulties, Veljković and Slavić[9] proposed the potential of a simplified analytical form which rather accurately reproduced the tabular values of the Heine–Abarenkov potential form-factor.[4] This model potential has the following form:

$$\langle \mathbf{k} + \mathbf{q}|\omega|\mathbf{k} \rangle = \beta_1 \frac{\sin(2\pi\beta_2\eta)}{2\pi\eta} \tag{10}$$

where η represents $q/2k_f$, and β_1 and β_2 are model parameters adjusted to the tabular values of the form-factor cited in Eq. (3). The values of these parameters are given in Table 1. Because of its simple form, this potential is suitable for practical use; however with the exception of its simplicity it has no other advantages over other potentials used up to the present time in the theory of metals.

In an effort to make the model potential described by Eq. (10) more general, one of the authors[10] tried to establish the correlation between parameters β_1 and β_2 and some general physical quantity. In studying various possibilities, he found that the relationship between these parameters and the atomic

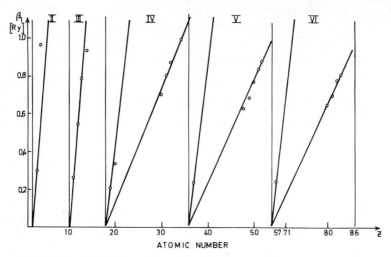

FIGURE 1   Periodic dependence of model parameter β_1 on atom number Z.

number is the most suitable one. Figures 1 and 2 show how the values of β_1 and β_2 change along the periodic system. As can be seen in the diagrams, the linear dependence which was discovered allows us to present the model parameters in the following form:

$$\beta_1 = \alpha_1 (Z - Z_0)$$

$$\beta_2 = \alpha_2 (Z - Z_0)$$

(11)

where Z is the atomic number of the metal under consideration, Z_0 the atomic number of the inert gas ending the previous period, while values of the coefficients of proportionality α_1 and α_2 are as follows:

$$\alpha_1 = \begin{cases} -0.2500 \text{ Ry} \\ \\ -0.0625 \text{ Ry} \end{cases} \qquad \alpha_2 = \begin{cases} 0.520 \text{ for short and for the first} \\ \text{half of long periods.} \\ 0.048 \text{ for the second half of long} \\ \text{periods.} \end{cases}$$

Eq. (11) shows that the value $(Z - Z_0)$ is nothing but the number of electrons outside the last closed shell of a given element. Hereafter we will refer to it as the quasi-valence number (QVN) and express it as Z^*. As can be readily seen, the QVN for elements of the first two short periods of the periodic table coincides with the usual Pauling valence. If this is taken into account, then Eq. (11) may be written as follows:

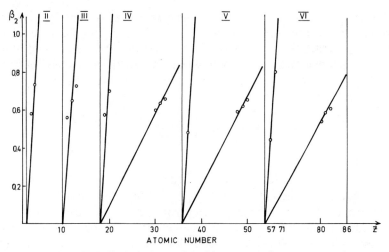

FIGURE 2   Periodic dependence of model parameter β_2 on atom number Z.

$$\beta_1 = \alpha_1 Z^*$$

$$\beta_2 = \alpha_2 Z^* \tag{12}$$

On the basis of Expressions (12), Eq. (10) may be expressed in the following manner:

$$\langle \mathbf{k} + \mathbf{q} | \omega | \mathbf{k} \rangle = \alpha_1 Z^* \frac{\sin (2\pi \alpha_2 Z^* \eta)}{2\pi \eta}. \tag{13}$$

The Fermi momentum k_F, which is introduced in Eq. (13) through the variable η, may also be presented, as already shown,[10] as a function dependent only upon Z^*:

$$k_F = (1.5\alpha_1 \alpha_2)^{1/2} Z^*. \tag{14}$$

After these corrections have been made, the arrived-at potential (13) becomes substantially different from all other phenomenological potentials used at present in the theory of metals. It is the only potential of a general nature without free parameters. For this reason it can also be applied to transition metals, whereas the majority of other potentials cannot be used in such a case.

The characteristics of the general model pseudopotential (13) mentioned above give it yet another considerable advantage over other potentials: it can be easily applied in analysing various characteristics of complex systems within the framework of the pseudoatomic approximation of Eq. (2). In this approximation, a complex system is treated as a homogeneous system composed of pseudoatoms bearing the averaged characteristics of atomic types out of which the analysed real system is composed. In considering this system, to apply Eq. (13) it is sufficient to determine the average QVN (AQVN) in the following way:

$$Z^*_{av} = \sum_{i=1}^{n} c_i Z_i^* \qquad (15)$$

where c_i is the concentration of the i-th component, Z_i^* the QVN of the i-th component, and n the number of components in the system.

On the basis of this simple pseudopotential, satisfactory results were obtained in the analysis of various characteristics of complex polymetallic systems, regardless of their highly complex nature. Success was noted in the treatment of the superconductivity of intermetallic compounds[11,12] and their formation heat,[13] the change of volume of polymetallic systems caused by diffusion,[14] the relation between the stability of intermetallic phases,[15] and the electrical resistance of complex metallic liquid systems,[16-17] etc. It is difficult to discuss the physical background of the important role played by the AQVN in describing phenomena in complex metallic systems. The results obtained so far allow us only to point out that this simple feature, the AQVN, is a decidedly important factor in defining the electronic properties of metals. Later we will see that it also plays a crucial role in determining the properties of biological systems.

Now let's consider the problem of chemical carcinogenesis. In view of the rôle played by the electron–ion interaction potential in condensed systems, we might expect its use to be of value in studying biological processes as well, since these processes are themselves the result of specific molecular interactions. We know from physics that such specific interactions are, in fact, based on the electron–ion potential but the relationship is not simple, and for reasons mentioned above, we are still incapable of dealing with it in an exact way for complex molecular systems without applying some crude approximations. To avoid this difficulty, we decided therefore to investigate the relationship between the electron–ion interaction potential for carcinogenic molecules and the ultimate effect of their carcinogenic action. This activity would result from the interaction of these carcinogenic molecules with macromolecules of DNA, RNA, or proteins in cells.

When it came to transferring this idea into real use, however, we were still faced with the problem of choosing an appropriate form for the potential. In view of the results achieved by potential (13) in the study of complex condensed systems, we decided to adapt it for this purpose. As its structure shows, it has four basic components: Coulomb's component derived from the nucleus charge, the screening of this component resulting from bound electrons, Pauli repulsion due to the interaction between conductive and bound electrons and, finally, the screening of free electrons. The last component characterizes the metal state and has to be eliminated in order to use the potential for the specified purpose. Eq. (2) shows that this is easily achievable if the potential (13) is multiplied by the dielectric function. To obtain the required potential in the configurational space we must also perform the inverse Fourier transform, as follows:

$$V(\mathbf{R}) = \frac{\Omega_0}{(2\pi)^3} \int\limits_0^\infty V(q) e^{-i\mathbf{q}\mathbf{R}} d^3 q. \tag{16}$$

In order to simplify this integration, the authors of Ref. 18 introduced an exponential prefactor into potential (13) which had the effect of enhancing the convergence of the integral in the region of large values of the change in momentum q. The potential modified in this way had the following form:

$$\langle \mathbf{k} + \mathbf{q} | \omega | \mathbf{k} \rangle = \alpha_1 Z^* \frac{\sin (2\pi\alpha_2 Z^* \eta)}{2\pi\eta} \exp (-\alpha_3 \eta). \tag{17}$$

The values of the coefficient $\mathbf{q}$ were determined so that the potential of Eq. (17) could give the most accurate values in the proximity of the point $q = 2k_F$. These are the most important terms in the study of electronic properties. The values thus determined are given by

$$\alpha_3 = \begin{cases} 0.3 \text{ for the first and second group in the periodic table.} \\ 0.4 \text{ for other groups of the periodic table.} \end{cases}$$

The second approximation relates to the screening function. Instead of the relatively complex Hartree dielectric function, we made use of the approximated expression

$$\varepsilon(q) = 1 + 2(D/\eta) \exp (-\eta/2) \tag{18}$$

where

$$D = \frac{1}{2\pi k_F R_0} \tag{19}$$

and R_0 is the Bohr radius.

The results for the effects of screening obtained by Eq. (18) differed by 5% from those obtained using Hartree's dielectric function; this may be considered satisfactory agreement for our purpose.

By integration of Eq. (16), we obtained the electron–free ion interaction potential in the configurational space. It has the following form:†

$$V(r) = Z^* e^2 / r - f(r) + F_1(r) \cdot F_2(r) \tag{20}$$

where

$$f(R) = \frac{e^2 \Omega_0}{(2\pi)^3 R_0} \alpha_1 \alpha_2 (Z - Z_0)^2 \left(\frac{4\pi\mu}{|\mu^2 + (b+R)^2||\mu^2 + (b-R)^2|} \right);$$

$$F_1(R) = \frac{e^2 \Omega_0}{(2\pi)^3 R_0^2} \cdot \frac{4}{\pi} \cdot \alpha_1 (Z - Z_0) \left(\frac{3\pi^2 Z^*}{\Omega_0} \right)^{2/3};$$

$$F_2(R) = \arctan\left(\frac{2\rho b}{b^2 - \rho^2 - R^2} \right) - \frac{b}{R} \arctan\left(\frac{2\rho R}{b^2 + \rho^2 - R^2} \right) -$$

$$- \frac{\rho}{2R} \left(\frac{\rho^2 + (b-R)^2}{\rho^2 + (b+R)^2} \right);$$

$$\mu = \frac{\alpha_3}{2} \left(\frac{\Omega_0}{3\pi^2 Z^*} \right)^{1/3}; \qquad \rho = \mu \left(1 + \frac{1}{2\alpha_3} \right);$$

$$b = \pi \alpha_2 (Z - Z_0)(\Omega_0 / 3\pi^2 Z^*)^{1/3}.$$

This potential could be applied to a molecule only within the framework of the pseudoatomic approximation. As in the case of intermetallic compounds, the molecule here is considered a homogeneous system composed of pseudoatoms bearing the averaged characteristics of real components of the molecule under consideration. The AQVN of such a system is represented by the expression

$$Z^*_{av} = \frac{\sum_{i=1}^{n} C_i Z_i}{N} \tag{21}$$

where Z_i^* is the QVN of the i-th component, C_i the number of atoms of the i-th component, n the number of components in the molecule, and N the total number of atoms in the molecule.

---

† In Eq. (20), α_1 is a dimensionless parameter.

To find some numerical characteristic which could allow us to follow the behaviour of individual organic agents in relation to their carcinogenic activity, it was decided to take the value of pseudopotential (20) at a distance of 5 Å. There was no particular physical reason for this choice; the decision was based upon an estimation that the region of intermolecular interactions was somewhere between 5 and 10 Å.

A number of organic compounds has been classified according to the value of their pseudopotentials, calculated in this manner. The results obtained demonstrated that with respect to the pseudopotential the analysed organic compounds could be divided into two groups; a group of potential carcinogens covering the range below -4.5 eV, and a group of noncarcinogens covering the range above this value.[19] Table 2 illustrates this result with a number of compounds.

The result obtained was clearly encouraging. In addition to its practical significance it opens up a new approach to the analysis of chemical carcinogenesis. The next step was to apply the electron–ion interaction potential to such an analysis more adequately.

After considering several possibilities, we opted to use the average value of the pseudopotential. Averaging was easier to conduct with potential (17) in its momentum representation because of its simpler analytical form, but the following question presented itself: over which limits should the averaging be computed? Since we did not have a more reliable physical criterion, we considered metals and intermetallic compounds, for which terms for values of η up to 1 radically affect the electronic properties. In selecting a lower limit for averaging, it was impossible to begin the integration from $\eta = 0$, since at this point potential (17) goes to infinity. After trials with different values for the lower limit, however, we came to the conclusion that the ultimate result was relatively independent of the choice of this limit; thus we opted for a lower η-value of 0.05. In the interval thus defined, the average value of the electron–ion interaction potential was established as follows:

$$W_{av}(q) = \frac{1}{0.95} \int\limits_{0.05}^{1} W^0(\eta) d\eta. \tag{22}$$

In this case it was not necessary to introduce the approximate screening function while performing the numerical integration. In our calculations Hartree's dielectric function was used. The results obtained using Eq. (22) are presented in Table 3 and by histogram in Figure 3 for 316 compounds from the IARC monographs.[2] Altogether there are 287 carcinogenic substances and of these, 202 organic carcinogens, *i.e.* 70.3% of all carcinogens considered, lie in the interval from 3.30 to 3.80 Ry.

TABLE 2

Correlation between potential strength and carcinogenicity of organic compounds.

Substance	Strength of potential, eV	Carcinogenicity
1,2-Diethylhydrazine	−2.9	+
Acetamide	−3.8	+
4-Aminoazobenzene	−3.8	+
Benzidine	−3.8	+
Norethisterone	−3.8	+
Benz(a)anthracene	−3.9	+
Benzo(b)fluoranthene	−3.9	+
Chrysene	−3.9	+
Diacetylaminoazotoluene	−3.9	+
Nitrosoethylurea	−4.2	+
Aflatoxin B1	−4.3	+
Aflatoxin G2	−4.3	+
β-Propiolactone	−4.3	+
Streptozotocin	−4.3	+
Amitrole	−4.5	+
Diazomethane	−4.5	+
1,3-Propane sultone	−4.5	+
5-Methylpropane	−4.5	+
Eosin disodium salt	−4.6	−
Orange I	−4.6	−
Ponceau MX	−4.7	−
4-Amino-2-nitrophenol	−4.8	−
Carmoisine	−4.9	−
5-Bromouracil	−4.9	−
2-Aminopurine	−4.9	−
Furylfuramide	−4.9	−
8-Azoguanine	−5.0	−
Orange G	−5.0	−
Sunset Yellow FCF	−5.0	−
Proflavine	−5.0	−
Hypoxanthine	−5.2	−
Amaranth	−5.2	−
Xanthine	−5.2	−
5-Nitro-2-furamidoxime	−5.6	−

If we consider the density of carcinogens per unit interval of 0.1 Ry within the interval of 3.30–3.80 Ry, we find that the average density of carcinogens per unit interval is 41.2. The average density of carcinogens per unit interval in the region beginning in the limits of 2.80 and 4.20 Ry, but excluding the above section (3.30–3.80 Ry), is 9.44. The ratio of these two densities is 4.36.

This clearly indicates a relationship between the carcinogenic activity of organic compounds and their electron–ion interaction potential. The number of noncarcinogenic agents for which data was available is much smaller, due to preselection of compounds covered by the IARC monographs. This point will be discussed in the next chapter. On the other hand, if we examine the

TABLE 3

Average potential values, average quasi-valence numbers, u.v.-absorption maxima, carcinogenic activity and types of tumours induced by organic compounds treated by the IARC (Ref. 1).

Substance	Formula	Z^*	$W(q)$, Ry	λ, nm	Carcinogen	Type of cancer†
Chlorinated hydrocarbons						
Carbon tetrachloride*	CCl_4	1.60	1.92		+	A
Chloroform*	$CHCl_3$	1.60	1.92		+	A
Aromatic amines						
Auramine	$C_{17}H_{21}N_3$	2.54	3.38		+	A, B, C
Benzidine*	$C_{12}H_{12}N$	2.69	3.51		+	A, C
4-Aminobiphenyl*	$C_{12}H_{11}N$	2.67	3.49		+	A, D
3,3'-Dimethylbenzidine (ortho-tolidine)*	$C_{14}H_{16}N_2$	2.56	3.39		+	
N-Nitroso compounds						
N-Nitrosodimethylamine*	$C_2H_6N_2O$	2.73	3.53	233	+	A, C, H
N-Nitrosodiethylamine*	$C_4H_{10}N_2O$	2.47	3.31	232	+	A, H
Nitrosomethylurea*	$C_2H_5N_3O_2$	3.33	3.93	231	+	C, H, N
Nitrosoethylurea*	$C_3H_7N_3O_2$	3.07	3.78	233	+	N, H
N-Methyl-N,4-dinitroso-aniline	$C_7H_7N_3O_2$	3.26	3.89		+	A, C, H
Natural products						
Aflatoxin B$_1$*	$C_{17}H_{12}O_6$	3.31	3.92	223	+	A
Aflatoxin B$_2$*	$C_{17}H_{12}O_6$	3.19	3.85	222	+	A
Aflatoxin G$_1$*	$C_{17}H_{12}O_7$	3.39	3.96	243	+	A
Aflatoxin M$_1$	$C_{17}H_{12}O_7$	3.39	3.96	226	+	A
Aflatoxin P$_1$	$C_{16}H_{10}O_6$	3.44	3.99	266	−	
Cycasin*	$C_8H_{16}N_2O_7$	3.03	3.76	218	+	A, C, H
Methylazoxymethanol acetate*	$C_4H_8N_2O_3$	3.06	3.78	215	+	A, C, H
Safrole*	$C_{10}H_{10}O_2$	2.82	3.60		+	A, H

Substance	Formula	Z^*	$W(q)$, Ry	λ, nm	Carcinogen	Type of cancer†
Isosafrole*	$C_{10}H_{10}O_2$	2.82	3.60		+	A, H
Dihydrosafrole*	$C_{10}H_{12}O_2$	2.67	3.49		+	A, H
Sterigmatocystin*	$C_{18}H_{12}O_6$	3.33	3.93	233	+	A, C
Miscellaneous						
N-[4-(5-Nitro-2-furyl)-2-thiazolyl]acetamide*	$C_9H_7O_4N_3S$	3.66	4.11	226	+	C, H
Polycyclic aromatic hydrocarbons						
Benz(a)anthracene*	$C_{18}H_{12}$	2.80	3.59		+	A, H, D
Benzo(b)fluoranthene*	$C_{20}H_{12}$	2.88	3.65		+	C, D
Benzo(j)fluoranthene*	$C_{20}H_{12}$	2.88	3.65		+	D
Benzo(a)pyrene*	$C_{20}H_{12}$	2.88	3.65		+	D
Benzo(e)pyrene	$C_{20}H_{12}$	2.88	3.65		+	D
Chrysene	$C_{18}H_{12}$	2.80	3.59		+	D
Benz(a,h)anthracene*	$C_{22}H_{14}$	2.83	3.61		+	C, D, H
Dibenzo(a,e)pyrene*	$C_{24}H_{14}$	2.89	3.66		+	C, D
Dibenzo(a,h)pyrene*	$C_{24}H_{14}$	2.89	3.66		+	C, D
Dibenzo(a,i)pyrene*	$C_{24}H_{14}$	2.89	3.66		+	C, D
Dibenzo(a,l)pyrene	$C_{24}H_{14}$	2.89	3.66		+	C
Indeno(1,2,3-cd)pyrene*	$C_{22}H_{12}$	2.94	3.69		+	D
Heterocyclic compounds						
Benz(c)acridine	$C_{17}H_{11}N$	2.90	3.67		+	D
Dibenz(a,h)acridine*	$C_{21}H_{13}N$	2.91	3.68		+	C, D
Dibenz(a,j)acridine*	$C_{21}H_{13}N$	2.91	3.68		+	C, H
7H-Dibenzo(c,g)carbazole*	$C_{20}H_{13}N$	2.88	3.65		+	A, C, D, H
Aromatic amines and related compounds						
Aniline	C_6H_7N	2.57	3.40		+	
3,3'-Dimethoxybenzidine*	$C_{14}H_{16}N_2O_2$	2.76	3.56		+	D
3,3'-Dichlorobenzidine*	$C_{12}H_{10}N_2Cl_2$	2.69	3.51		+	D
para-Magenta	$C_{19}H_{17}N_3Cl$	2.72	3.52		+	C

4,4'-Methylene bis(2-chloraniline)*	$C_{13}H_{12}N_2Cl_2$	2.62	3.45		+	A, H
4,4'-Methylene bis(2-methylaniline)*	$C_{15}H_{18}N_2$	2.51	3.35		+	A
4,4'-Methylenedianiline	$C_{18}H_{14}N_2$	2.62	3.45		+	A
1-Naphthylamine	$C_{10}H_9N$	2.70	3.51		+	A, C
2-Naphthylamine*	$C_{10}H_9N$	2.70	3.51		+	A, D
4-Nitrobiphenyl	$C_{12}H_9NO_2$	3.08	3.79		+	
N,N-bis(2-Chloroethyl)-2-naphthylamine	$C_{14}H_{16}Cl_2N$	2.44	3.29		+	
Hydrazine and derivatives						
1,1-Dimethylhydrazine*	$C_2H_8N_2$	2.17	3.03		+	C, A
1,2-Dimethylhydrazine*	$C_2H_8N_2$	2.17	3.03		+	C, H
1,2-Diethylhydrazine*	$C_4H_{12}N_2$	2.11	2.97		+	
Isonicotinic acid hydrazide	$C_6H_7N_3O$	3.06	3.78		+	H
Maleic hydrazide	$C_4H_4N_2O$	3.50	4.02		−	
N-Nitroso compounds						
N-Methyl-N'-nitro-N-nitrosoguanidine*	$C_2H_5N_5O_3$	3.73	4.13	275	+	C, H
N-Nitroso-di-n-butylamine	$C_8H_{18}N_2O$	2.28	3.14	233	+	D, H
N-Nitroso-N-methylurethane*	$C_4H_8N_2O_3$	3.06	3.78	237	+	D, H
Streptozotocin*	$C_8H_{15}N_3O_7$	3.15	3.83	228	+	C, H
Miscellaneous alkylating agents						
bis(Chloromethyl ether)*	$C_2H_4Cl_2O$	2.22	3.08		+	
Chloromethyl methyl ether*	C_2H_5ClO	2.22	3.08		+	
1,4-Butanediol dimethane sulphonate	$C_6H_{14}O_6S_2$	3.07	3.78		+	C
1,3-Propane sultone*	$C_3H_6O_3S$	3.23	3.88		+	C, H, N
β-Propiolactone*	$C_3H_4O_2$	3.11	3.81		+	
Dimethyl sulphate*	$C_2H_6O_4S$	3.38	3.96		+	N
Diethyl sulphate*	$C_4H_{10}O_4S$	2.95	3.71		+	D

Substance	Formula	Z^*	$W(q)$, Ry	λ, nm	Carcinogen	Type of cancer†
Some organochlorine pesticides						
Aldrin	$C_{12}H_8Cl_6$	2.38	3.23		+	C, H
Aramite*	$C_{12}H_{23}ClO_4S$	2.50	3.34		+	A, H
Lindane*	$C_6H_6Cl_6$	2.00	2.84		+	A
Chlorobenzilate	$C_{16}H_{14}Cl_2O_3$	2.80	3.59		+	A
DDT*	$C_{14}H_9Cl_5$	2.50	3.34		+	A, H
TDE (DDD)	$C_{14}H_{10}Cl_4$	2.50	3.34		+	A
Dieldrin*	$C_{12}H_8Cl_6O$	2.57	3.40		+	A, H
Endrin	$C_{12}H_8Cl_6O$	2.52	3.36		+	
Heptachlor	$C_{10}H_5Cl_7$	2.36	3.21		+	A
Heptachlor epoxide	$C_{10}H_5Cl_7O$	2.52	3.36		+	A
Methoxychlor	$C_{16}H_{15}Cl_3O_2$	2.61	3.44		+	H
Mirex*	$C_{10}H_{12}$	2.36	3.21		+	A
Quintozene (pentachloro-nitrobenzene)	$C_6Cl_5NO_2$	3.28	3.90		+	A
Sex hormones						
Diethylstilbestrol (stilbestrol)*	$C_{18}H_{20}O_2$	2.60	3.43		+	
Ethinyloestradiol*	$C_{20}H_{24}O_2$	2.52	3.36	248	+	
Mestranol*	$C_{21}H_{26}O_2$	2.49	3.33	225	+	
Oestradiol-17β*	$C_{18}H_{25}O_2$	2.46	3.30	280	+	
Oestriol	$C_{18}H_{24}O_3$	2.53	3.37	283	+	
Oestrone*	$C_{18}H_{24}O_3$	2.53	3.37	240	+	
Progesterone	$C_{21}H_{30}O_2$	2.38	3.23	240	+?	
Chloromadinone acetate	$C_{23}H_{29}ClO_4$	2.56	3.39	283	+?	
Medroxyprogesterone acetate	$C_{24}H_{34}O_4$	2.48	3.32	240	+	
Dimethisterone	$C_{23}H_{32}O_2$	2.39	3.97	240	+?	
Ethynodiol diacetate	$C_{24}H_{32}O_4$	2.53	3.37		+	
Norethisterone	$C_{20}H_{26}O_2$	2.46	3.30	240	+	
Norethisterone acetate	$C_{22}H_{28}O_3$	2.53	3.37	240	+	
Norethynodrel	$C_{20}H_{26}O_2$	2.46	3.30		+	

Norgestrel	$C_{21}H_{28}O_2$	2.43	3.28		+?	
Testosterone*	$C_{19}H_{28}O_2$	2.37	3.22	238	+	
Anti-thyroid and related substances						
Amitrole*	$C_2H_4N_4$	3.20	3.86		+	A, H
Ethylenethiourea*	$C_3H_6N_2S$	2.83	3.61		+	A
Methylthiouracil*	$C_5H_6N_2OS$	3.20	3.86	214	+	H
Propylthiouracil*	$C_7H_{10}N_2OS$	2.86	3.64	214	+	H
Thioacetamide*	C_2H_5NS	2.67	3.49	210	+	H
Thiouracil	$C_4H_4N_2OS$	3.50	4.02	212	+	A, H
Thiourea*	CH_4N_2S	3.00	3.74	241	+	H
Urethane*	$C_3H_7NO_2$	2.77	3.56		+	A, C, H
2-Amino-5-(5-nitro-2-furyl)-1,3,4-thiadiazole*	$C_6H_4N_4O_3S$	4.00	4.24	287	+	D
2-(2-Formylhydrazine)-4-(5-nitro-2-furyl)thiazole*	$C_8H_6N_4O_4S$	3.82	4.17	385	+	H
5-(Morpholinomethyl)-3-[(nitrofurfurylidene)amino]-2-oxazolidinone*	$C_{13}H_{16}N_4O_6$	3.18	3.85	258	+	
5-(Morpholinomethyl)-3-[(nitrofurfurylidene)amino]-2-oxazolidinone tartarate	$C_{17}H_{22}N_4O_{12}$	3.31	3.92	258	–	
5-Nitro-2-furaldehyde semicarbazone	$C_6H_6N_4O_4$	3.70	4.12	260	–	
1-[(5-Nitrofurfurylidene)amino]-2-imidiazolidinone*	$C_8H_8N_4O_4$	3.50	4.02	257	+	
Acetamide	C_2H_5NO	2.67	3.49	250	+	A, H
Benzene*	C_6H_6	2.50	3.34		+	
Diazomethane	CH_2N_2	3.22	3.87		+	
ortho-Dichlorobenzene	$C_6H_4Cl_2$	2.50	3.34		+?	
para-Dichlorobenzene	$C_6H_4Cl_2$	2.50	3.34		+?	
Ethyl methanesulphonate*	$C_3H_8O_3S$	2.93	3.69		+	
Methyl methanesulphonate*	$C_2H_6O_3S$	3.17	3.84		+	N
Polychlorinated biphenyls*	$C_{12}X_{10}$	2.63	3.46		+	A, H
Vinyl chloride*	C_2H_3Cl	2.00	2.84		+	

Some aromatic azo compounds

Substance	Formula	Z^*	$W(q)$, Ry	λ, nm	Carcinogen	Type of cancer†
Amaranth	$C_{20}H_{11}N_2Na_3O_{10}S_3$	3.71	4.12	520	–	
para-Aminoazobenzene	$C_{12}H_{11}N_3$	2.85	3.63		+	A
ortho-Aminoazobenzene	$C_{12}H_{11}N_3$	2.85	3.63		+	A, D, H
ortho-Aminoazotoluene*	$C_{14}H_{15}N_3$	2.69	3.51	326	+	A
Azobenzene	$C_{12}H_{10}N_2$	2.83	3.61		–	
Carmoisine	$C_{20}H_{12}N_2Na_2O_7S_2$	3.51	3.35		+	A, C
Chrysoidine	$C_{12}H_{13}ClN_4$	2.73	3.53		+	
C.I. Disperse Yellow 3	$C_{15}H_{15}N_3O_2$	3.00	3.74		+	C, H
Citrus Red No. 2*	$C_{18}H_{16}N_2O_3$	2.97	3.72		–	
D & C Red No. 9	$C_{17}H_{13}ClN_2O_4BaS_{1/2}$	3.14	3.82	487	+	A
Diacetylaminoazotoluene	$C_{18}H_{19}N_3O_2$	2.81	3.60		+	
2,6-Diamino-3-(phenylazo)-pyridine	$C_{11}H_{11}N_5$	2.96	3.71	238	+	A
para-Dimethylaminoazo-benzene*	$C_{14}H_{15}N_3$	2.69	3.51		+	A
para-Dimethylaminobenzene-diazosodium sulphonate	$C_8H_{10}N_3NaO_3S$	3.15	3.83		+	A
Evans Blue	$C_{34}H_{24}N_6Na_4O_{14}S_4$	3.45	4.00	490	+	C
4-Hydroxyazobenzene	$C_{12}H_{10}N_2O$	2.96	3.71	492	+	D
Methyl Red	$C_{15}H_{15}N_3O_2$	3.00	3.74	476	+	
Oil Orange SS*	$C_{17}H_{14}N_2O$	2.88	3.65	474	–	
Orange I	$C_{16}H_{11}N_2NaO_4S$	3.31	3.92	506	–	
Orange G	$C_{16}H_{10}N_2Na_2O_7S_2$	3.59	4.06	508	–	
Ponceau MX*	$C_{18}H_{14}N_2Na_2O_7S$	3.38	3.96	500	+	D, H
Ponceau 3R*	$C_{19}H_{16}N_2Na_2O_7S_2$	3.29	3.91		+	A, H
Ponceau SX	$C_{18}H_{14}N_2Na_2O_7S_2$	3.38	3.96		–	
Scarlet Red	$C_{24}H_{20}N_4O$	2.90	3.67		+	A
Sudan I	$C_{16}H_{12}N_2O$	2.97	3.72	514	+	
Sudan II	$C_{18}H_{16}N_2O$	2.81	3.60	492	–	
Sudan III	$C_{22}H_{16}N_4O$	3.02	3.75		+	D
Sudan Brown RR	$C_{16}H_{14}N_4$	2.88	3.65		+	C, H

Name	Formula					
Sunset Yellow FCF	$C_{16}H_{10}N_2Na_2O_7S_2$	3.59	3.42	480	−	C
Trypan Blue*	$C_{34}H_{24}N_6Na_4O_{14}S_4$	3.51	3.35	584	+	
Yellow AB	$C_{16}H_{13}N_3$	2.88	3.65	434	−	
Yellow OB	$C_{17}H_{15}N_3$	2.80	3.59	436	−	
Aziridines						
Aphalate	$C_{12}H_{24}N_9P_3$	2.75	3.55		−	
Aziridine	C_2H_5N	2.25	3.11		+	A
2-(1-Aziridinyl)ethanol	C_4H_9NO	2.40	3.25		+	
Aziridyl benzoquinone	$C_{16}H_{22}N_2O_6$	2.87	3.64		+	
bis(1-Aziridinyl)morpho-linophosphine sulphide	$C_8H_{16}N_3POS$	2.67	3.49			
2-Methylaziridine*	C_3H_7N	2.18	3.04		+	H
tris(Aziridinyl)-para-benzoquinone	$C_{12}H_{13}N_3O_2$	2.93	3.69		+	C, H
tris(1-Aziridinyl) phosphine oxide	$C_6H_{12}N_3PO$	2.70	3.51		+	A, C, H
tris(1-Aziridinyl) phosphine sulphide*	$C_6H_{12}N_3PS$	2.70	3.51		+	H
2,4,6-tris(1-Aziridinyl)-s-triazine	$C_9H_{12}N_6$	2.89	3.66	226	+	D, H
tris(2-Methyl-1-aziri-dinyl)phosphine oxide	$C_9H_{18}N_3OP$	2.50	3.34		+	
Mustards						
bis(2-Chloroethyl) ether	$C_4H_8Cl_2O$	2.13	2.99		+	
Chlorambucil*	$C_{14}H_{19}Cl_2NO_2$	2.47	3.31	258	+	A, H
Cyclophosphamide*	$C_7H_{15}Cl_2N_2PO_2$	2.48	3.32		+	D, H
Mannomustine	$C_{10}H_{22}Cl_2N_2O_4$	2.45	3.29		+	C, H
Melphalan*	$C_{13}H_{18}Cl_2N_2O_2$	2.54	3.38	260	+	
Mustard gas*	$C_4H_8Cl_2S$	2.13	2.99		+	D, H
Nitrogen mustard*	$C_5H_{11}Cl_2N$	2.00	2.84		+	
Nitrogen mustard N-oxide*	$C_5H_{11}Cl_2NO$	2.20	3.06		+	
Oestradiol mustard	$C_{42}H_{50}Cl_4N_2O_4$	2.51	3.35	261	+	
Phenoxybenzamine	$C_{18}H_{22}ClNO$	2.17	3.03	272	+	
Trichlorotriethylamine	$C_6H_{12}Cl_3NO$	2.00	2.84		+	
Uracil mustard*	$C_8H_{11}Cl_2N_3O_2$	2.77	3.56	257	+	

B

Substance	Formula	Z^*	$W(g)$, Ry	λ, nm	Carcinogen	Type of cancer†
Some naturally occurring substances						
Actinomycin D*	$C_{62}H_{86}N_{12}O_{16}$	2.78	3.57	240	+	
Adriamycin	$C_{27}H_{29}NO_{11}$	3.10	3.80	233	+	
Azaserine*	$C_5H_7N_3O_4$	3.47	4.00	252	+	
Canthardin	$C_{10}H_{12}O_4$	2.92	3.68		+	
Chloramphenicol*	$C_{11}H_{12}Cl_2N_2O_5$	3.06	3.78	278	+	
Cholesterol	$C_{27}H_{46}O$	2.16	3.02		+	H
Coumarin	$C_9H_6O_2$	3.18	3.85	209	+	H
Cyclochloratine	$C_{24}H_{31}Cl_2N_5O_7$	2.84	3.62	257	+	A
Daunomycin*	$C_{27}H_{29}NO_{10}$	3.01	3.75	234	+	C
Griseofulvin	$C_{17}H_{17}ClO_6$	2.98	3.73	286	+	A
Luteoskyrin	$C_{30}H_{22}O_{12}$	3.34	3.93	280	+	H
Mitomycin C*	$C_{15}H_{18}N_4O_5$	3.05	3.77	216	+	
Ochratoxin A	$C_{20}H_{18}ClNO_6$	3.04	3.76	215	+	
Parascorbic acid	$C_6H_8O_2$	2.75	3.55		+	H
Patulin	$C_7H_6O_4$	3.41	3.98		+	
Penicillic acid	$C_8H_{10}O_4$	3.00	3.74	220	+	
Reserpine	$C_{33}H_{40}N_2O_3$	2.81	3.60	216	+	A, C
Tannic acid	$C_7H_6O_5$	3.56	4.04		+	
Pyrrolizidine alkaloids						
Hydroxysenkirkine	$C_{19}H_{27}NO_7$	2.78	3.57	217	+	
Jacobine	$C_{18}H_{25}NO_6$	2.76	3.56		+	
Lasiocarpine*	$C_{21}H_{33}NO_7$	2.65	3.48		+	
Monocrotaline*	$C_{16}H_{23}NO_6$	2.78	3.57		+	
Retrorsine	$C_{18}H_{25}NO_6$	2.76	3.56	217	+	A
Riddelline	$C_{18}H_{23}NO_6$	2.83	3.61		+?	
Seneciphylline	$C_{18}H_{23}NO_5$	2.77	3.56	281	–?	
Senkirkine	$C_{19}H_{27}NO_6$	2.72	3.52	215	+?	

Epoxides							
Diglycidyl resorcinol ether	$C_{12}H_{14}O_4$	2.87	3.64			+	
Epichlorohydrin*	C_3H_5ClO	2.40	3.25		+	+	
1-Epoxyethyl-3,4-epoxy-cyclohexane	$C_8H_{12}O_2$	2.53	3.37		+	+	
3,4-Epoxy-6-methylcyclo-hexylmethyl-3,4-epoxy-6-methylcyclohexane carboxylate	$C_{16}H_{24}O_4$	2.55	3.39			+	
cis-9,10-Epoxystearic acid	$C_{18}H_{34}O_3$	2.25	3.11			−?	
Ethylene oxide	C_2H_4O	2.57	3.40			−?	
Fusarenon-X	$C_{17}H_{22}O_8$	2.94	3.69	220	+	+	A
Glyceraldehyde*	$C_3H_4O_2$	3.11	3.81		+	+	
Glycidyl oleate	$C_{21}H_{38}O_3$	2.26	3.12		+	+	
Glycidyl stearate	$C_{21}H_{40}O_3$	2.22	3.08		+	+	
Propylene oxide	C_3H_6O	2.40	3.25		+	+	
Styrene oxide	C_8H_8O	2.71	3.52	250	+	+	
Triethylene glycol diglycidyl ether	$C_{12}H_{22}O_6$	2.65	3.48		+	+	
Miscellaneous industrial chemicals							
Benzyl chloride	C_7H_7Cl	2.40	3.25	217	+	+	
γ-Butyrolactone	$C_4H_6O_2$	2.83	3.61		+	+	
β-Butyrolactone*	$C_4H_6O_2$	2.83	3.61	209	+	−	A
Dinitrosopentamethylene-tetramine	$C_5H_{10}N_6O_2$	3.13	3.82			−	
1,4-Dioxane*	$C_4H_8O_2$	2.57	3.40	258	+	+	A, H
Ethylene sulphide	C_2H_4S	2.57	3.40		+	+	
Trichloroethylene	C_2HCl_3	2.00	2.84	230	+	+	
4-Vinylcyclohexane	C_8H_{12}	2.20	3.06		+	+	
Some carbamates, thiocarbamates and carbazides							
Carbaryl	$C_{12}H_{11}NO_2$	3.00	3.74		+	+	C
Chloropropham	$C_{10}H_{12}ClNO_2$	2.69	3.51		+	+	
Diallate	$C_{10}H_{17}Cl_2NOS$	2.38	3.23		+	+	A, H
Dimethylcarbamoyl chloride*	C_3H_6ClNO	2.50	3.34		+	+	

Substance	Formula	Z^*	$W(q)$, Ry	λ, nm	Carcinogen	Type of cancer†
Disulphiram	$C_{10}H_{20}N_2S_4$	2.61	3.44		+	A, C, H
Dulcin	$C_9H_{12}N_2O_2$	2.80	3.59	242	+	A
Ethyl selenac	$C_{20}H_{40}N_4S_8Se$	2.66	3.48		+	A, C
Ethyl tellurac	$C_{20}H_{40}N_4S_8Te$	2.66	3.48		+	
Ferbam	$C_9H_{18}FeN_3S_6$	3.05	3.77		+	
Ledate	$C_6H_{12}N_2PbS_4$	2.96	3.71		+	C
Methyl carbamate	$C_2H_5NO_2$	3.00	3.74		+	
Methyl selenac	$C_{12}H_{24}N_4S_8Se$	2.98	3.73		+	C
Manuron	$C_9H_{11}ClN_2O$	2.67	3.49	247	+	A, C, H
Phenicarbazide	$C_7H_9N_3O$	2.90	3.67	233	+	H
Potassium bis(2-hydroxy-ethyl)dithiocarbamate	$C_5H_{10}KNO_2S_2$	2.86	3.64		+	A
Propham	$C_{10}H_{13}NO_2$	2.69	3.51	236	+	
n-Propyl carbamate	$C_4H_9NO_2$	2.63	3.46		+	
Semicarbazide	CH_6ClN_3O	2.67	3.49	278	+	C
Sodium diethyldithio-carbamate	$C_5H_{10}NNaS_2$	2.53	3.37	257	+	A, H
Thiram	$C_6H_{12}N_2S_4$	2.92	3.68	243	+	A, H
Zectran	$C_{12}H_{18}N_2O_2$	2.55	3.39		+	H
Zineb	$C_4H_6N_2S_4Zn$	3.41	3.98		+	A, C, H
Ziram	$C_6H_{12}N_2S_4Zn$	2.88	4.19		+	
Some miscellaneous pharmaceutical substances						
Acriflavinium chloride	$C_{14}H_{14}N_3Cl$	2.69	3.51	261	+	
Aurothioglucose	$C_6H_{11}AuO_5S$	3.00	3.74		+	
Chloroquinone	$C_{18}H_{26}ClN_3$	2.38	3.23	220	+?	
Diazepam	$C_{16}H_{13}ClN_2O$	2.85	3.63	242	+	
Oxazepam*	$C_{15}H_{11}ClN_2O_2$	2.80	3.59	230	+	H
Dithranol	$C_{14}H_{10}O_3$	3.00	3.74	256	+	
Ethionamide	$C_8H_{10}N_2S$	2.76	3.56	290	+	
Hycanthone	$C_{20}H_{24}N_2O_2S$	2.69	3.51	233	+	
Hycanthone mesylate	$C_{21}H_{28}N_2O_5S_2$	2.83	3.61	232	+	
	$C_{?}H_{?}NO$	3.00	3.74	243	+	

Compound	Formula					
Metronidazole	$C_6H_9N_3O_3$	3.14	3.82	370	+	H
Niridazole*	$C_6H_6N_4O_3S$	3.70	4.12	250	+	H
Phenacetin*	$C_{10}H_{13}NO_2$	2.69	3.51	257	+	A
Phenobarbital*	$C_{12}H_{12}N_2O_3$	3.03	3.76		+	
Phenobarbital sodium*	$C_{12}H_{11}NaN_2O_3$	3.03	3.76		+	
Phenylbutazone	$C_{19}H_{20}N_2O_2$	2.74	3.54	239	+	
Oxyphenobutazone	$C_{19}H_{20}N_2O_3$	2.82	3.60	254	+	
Phenytoin*	$C_{15}H_{12}N_2O_2$	3.03	3.76	258	+	
Phenytoin sodium*	$C_{15}H_{11}NaN_2O_2$	3.03	3.76		+	
Pronetalol	$C_{15}H_9NO$	2.41	3.26		+	
Pyrimethamine	$C_{12}H_{13}ClN_4$	2.73	3.56		+	
Some fumigants, the herbicides 2,4-D and 2,4,5-T, chlorinated dibenzodioxins and miscellaneous compounds						
1,2-bis(Chloromethoxy)ethane	$C_4H_8Cl_2O$	2.73	3.56		+	
1,4-bis(Chloromethoxy-methol)benzene	$C_{10}H_{12}Cl_2O_2$	2.54	3.38		+	
Chlorinated dibenzodioxins	$C_{12}H_8(X_8)O_2$	3.09	3.79	228–260	+	C
Copper 8-hydroxyquinoline	$C_{18}H_{12}CuN_2O_2$	3.06	3.77		+	
2,4-Dichlorophenoxyacetic acid	$C_8H_6Cl_2O_3$	3.05	3.78		+	
1,2-Dibromo-3-chloro-propane*	C_3H_5BrCl	1.82	2.48		+	
trans-1,4-Dichlorobutene	$C_4H_6Cl_2$	2.00	2.84		+	
Catechol	$C_6H_6O_2$	3.00	3.74		+	
Resorcinol	$C_6H_6O_2$	3.00	3.74	214	+	
Hydroquinone	$C_6H_6O_2$	3.00	3.74	220	+	
Dimethoxane	$C_8H_{14}O_4$	2.69	3.51	228	+	A
Eosin	$C_{20}H_8Br_4O_5$	3.30	3.91	520	–	
Eosin disodium salt	$C_{20}H_6Br_4Na_2O_5$	3.30	3.91	519	–	
Ethylene dibromide*	$C_2H_4Br_2$	1.75	2.34		+	
Hexamethylphosphoramide*	$C_6H_{18}N_3PO$	2.34	3.20		–	
Isopropyl alcohol	C_3H_8O	2.17	3.03	181	+	C
Methyl iodide*	CH_3I	1.60	1.92		+	
para-Quinone	$C_6H_4O_2$	3.33	3.93		+	
Succinic anhydride	$C_4H_4O_3$	3.45	4.00	278	–?	
2,4,5-Trichlorophenoxy-acetic acid	$C_8H_5Cl_3O_3$	3.05	3.77	206	+	

Substance	Formula	Z^*	$W(q)$, Ry	λ, nm	Carcinogen	Type of cancer†
Hair dyes						
4-Amino-2-nitrophenol	$C_6H_6N_2O_3$	3.41	3.98	234	+	
2,4-Diaminoanisole	$C_7H_{10}N_2O$	2.70	3.51	511	−	
1,2-Diamino-4-nitro-benzene	$C_6H_7N_3O_2$	3.22	3.87	380	−	
1,4-Diamino-2-nitro-benzene	$C_6H_7N_3O$	3.22	3.87		−	
2,4-Diaminotoluene*	$C_7H_{10}N_2$	2.53	3.37	294	+	A
2,5-Diaminotoluene	$C_7H_{10}N_2$	2.53	3.37		+	
meta-Phenylenediamine	$C_6H_8N_2$	2.63	3.46	240	+	
para-Phenylenediamine	$C_6H_8N_2$	2.63	3.46	246	+?	
Colouring agents						
Benzyl Violet 4B*	$C_{38}H_{40}NaN_3O_6S_2$	2.86	3.64		+	C
Acridine Orange	$C_{17}H_{19}N_3$	2.62	3.45	490	−	
Blue VRS	$C_{27}H_{31}NaN_2O_6S_2$	2.87	3.65		+	
Brilliant Blue FCF	$C_{37}H_{34}N_2O_9S_3$	3.11	3.81		+	C
Fast Green FCF	$C_{37}H_{34}Na_2N_2O_{10}S_3$	3.09	3.79	628	+	C
Guinea Green B	$C_{37}H_{35}NaN_2O_6S_2$	2.95	3.71		+	A
Light Green SF	$C_{37}H_{34}Na_2N_2O_9S_3$	3.06	3.78		+	
Rhodamine B	$C_{28}H_{31}ClN_2O_3$	2.65	3.48	546	+	
Rhodamine 6G	$C_{28}H_{30}N_2O_3$	2.70	3.51	535	+	
Miscellaneous industrial chemicals						
5-Aminoacenaphthene	$C_{12}H_{11}N$	2.67	3.49	240	+	
Anthranilic acid	$C_7H_7NO_2$	3.06	3.78	217	+	
para-Chloro-ortho-toluidine	C_7H_8ClN	2.47	3.31	242	+	C
Cinnamyl anthraniliate	$C_{16}H_{15}NO_2$	2.82	3.60		+	
N,N'-Diacetylbenzidine*	$C_{16}H_{16}N_2O_2$	2.83	3.61		+	
4,4'-Diaminodiphenyl ether*	$C_{12}H_{12}N_2O$	2.81	3.60	293	+	C, H

3,3'-Dichloro-4,4'-diamino-diphenyl ether*	$C_{12}H_{10}Cl_2N_2O$	2.81	3.60		+	
2,4'-Diphenyldiamine	$C_{12}H_{12}N_2$	2.69	3.51	235	+	
5-Nitroacenaphthene*	$C_{12}H_9NO_2$	3.08	3.79	262	+	H
N-Phenyl-2-naphthylamine*	$C_{16}H_{13}N$	3.00	3.74		+	A
4,4'-Thiodianiline	$C_{12}H_{12}N_2S$	2.81	3.60		+	
ortho-Toluidine	C_7H_9N	2.47	3.31	232	+	
2,4-Xylidine	$C_8H_{11}N$	2.40	3.25	290	+	A, C
2,5-Xylidine	$C_8H_{11}N$	2.40	3.25	236	+	C

† A — Hepatoma, C — sarcoma, D — papilloma, H — adenocarcinoma.
* Carcinogens according to IARC criteria.

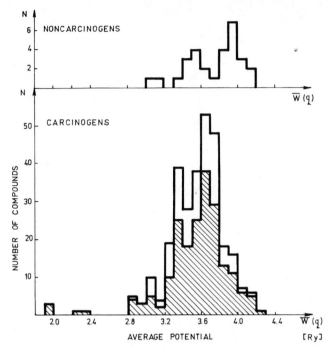

FIGURE 3 Distribution, with respect to their electron–ion interaction potentials, of carcinogenic and noncarcinogenic agents[2] (carcinogens according to IARC criteria are shaded).[2a]

distribution of these noncarcinogenic agents in terms of their potential, we see that there is no particular range in which their density would be considered higher. We can notice some shift in the potential corresponding to non-carcinogens, with respect to carginogens. This is shown in Figure 4.

If we use these results for the preselection of chemical compounds, the following conclusion may be made: If we have N randomly selected organic substances containing n carcinogens, on the basis of relation (22) we may estimate that about 70% of them will have their electron–ion interaction potential in the range between 3.30 and 3.80 Ry. When we apply this finding to compounds with unknown carcinogenic activity, we may conclude the following: If their potentials according to Eq. (22) are within the above-mentioned limits, the probability of their being carcinogenic is 4.36 times higher than if their average potentials fall outside this interval.

Some obvious objections might be raised with regard to this analysis, since it does not take into account the effects of structural isomerism and metabolic transformations of primary substances. This problem will be discussed in greater detail in the following chapter. For now we wish to point out that even without correction the existence of a correlation between the electron–ion

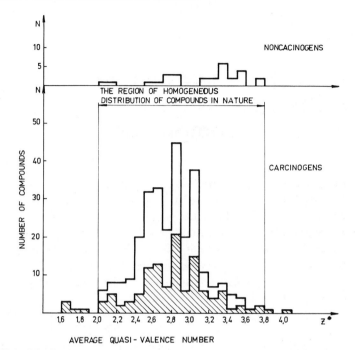

FIGURE 4   Distribution, with respect to their average quasi-valence numbers, of carcinogenic
and noncarcinogenic agents[2] (carcinogens according to IARC criteria are shaded).[2a]

interaction potential of organic compounds and their carcinogenic activity
cannot be questioned.

The results that we have obtained demonstrate that this analysis offers a
new approach to the study of chemical carcinogenesis. Explored at the level of
molecular interaction, this analysis may yield useful results, despite some
rough approximations. Moreover, the established correlation has some
practical meaning: it can be used as a preselection criterion when it is necessary
to determine the order of priorities in the study of chemical agents with respect
to their carcinogenicity. This becomes important in those particular cases
which often crop up in practice, when the number of agents greatly exceeds the
available experimental resources. Moreover, we should bear in mind that this
is a theoretical criterion. Preselection based upon it could be performed very
quickly and at little cost. Such preselection could reduce dependence on
mammalian tests, which are both expensive and time consuming, although still
unreplaceable.

CHAPTER 3

The Correlation Between the AQVN and the Carcinogenic Activity of Organic Compounds

We will now consider in more detail the interdependence of the pseudopotential described by Eq. (13) with the valence number, since the latter influences the former to a great extent. There are many other model pseudopotentials[3,4] which describe the electron–ion interaction quite sufficiently, but all contain two or more model parameters which must be determined in order for them to fit experimental data for every system analysed. The area of their application, then, is considerably reduced, particularly in the case of polycomponent systems. This problem does not exist, however, when working with pseudopotential (13) for it has no free parameters, and consists of no more than a function of the quasi-valence (atomic) number and the change of momentum. It is therefore different from all other pseudopotentials used at present in the theory of condensed matter.

The average quasi-valence number, which basically defines pseudopotential (13), represents the fundamental characteristic of every condensed system. Nonetheless its simple nature and the method of its determination, which is still simpler, make it seem too trivial a parameter to be taken seriously into account when considering any complex phenomenon within the framework of the existing theory of condensed matter. The successful results obtained by applying pseudopotential (13) in calculating a large number of various properties[12–17] demonstrate that such a view is misdirected, however.

The importance of the quasi-valence number in determining complex physical properties will be demonstrated by two characteristic examples. The first is related to the critical temperature (T_c) of the superconductive phase transition. This value is a function of a number of complex physical quantities of the system. This is also the reason why the critical temperature has yet to be exactly determined on the basis of first principles: existing theories do not allow for an exact treatment of complex polymetallic systems. The correlation between the valence number and critical temperature, on the other hand, was established two decades ago by analysis of experimental results. The phenomenological rule, known as the Matthias rule,[20] allows us to envisage with great certainty a system with n components having good superconductive characteristics. Despite numerous attempts over the past years, however, the contemporary theory of metals has not succeeded in fully reproducing these phenomenological results.

The second example deals with the correlation between the valence number and Fermi's energy. The latter, which largely determines numerous properties of metallic systems, is contingent upon a number of complex factors, such as the structure of the crystal lattice of a given system, ion structure, the type and strength of chemical bonds in a system, etc. Some of these characteristics of transition metals and their alloys cannot be described adequately by the solid state theory at its present-day level; therefore Fermi's energy in condensed systems cannot be calculated with sufficient accuracy. On the other hand, if pseudopotential (13) is taken as a starting point, this physical quantity can be expressed as a function of the valence number by the following simple relation:[10]

$$E_F = C \cdot Z^{*2}$$

where C is a proportionality coefficient independent of the nature of a specific system.

The correlation between pseudopotential (13) and carcinogenicity discussed earlier on the one hand, and the obvious role which the quasi-valence number plays in defining a series of complex characteristics of condensed systems on the other, prompted us to undertake a study of the correlation between carcinogenic properties of organic substances and their quasi-valence numbers (Z^*), despite the complexity of the various problems involved.

Before presenting the results of that study, we will first consider in some detail the experimental data used to establish this correlation. Selection of experimental data is not a simple task if one considers the great variety of biological experiments available and takes into account the theories on which they are based, the experimental techniques used, and the types of systems concerned. One of our principal selection criteria was the inclusion of metabolic transformations in substances tested. Later we will consider at greater length the problems associated with metabolic transformations of chemical substances.

Of all tests currently available, experimentation with mammalian systems has proved to be the most reliable. This is because during *in vitro* testing the agent under study is exposed to conditions which are closest to those existing in the human organism. For this reason our analysis was based upon results obtained from such testing.

The primary source of experimental data we used came from IARC monographs published in Lyon, France. These publications contain data on the carcinogenicity of various chemical compounds grouped according to type and method of application to animals. It is important to note that this data constitutes all studies of the activity of individual agents which have been published or in some other way communicated to the scientific community prior to the monographs' publication. In view of the large number of compounds covered, these monographs serve as an excellent basis for studying the connection(s) between physical and/or chemical parameters and the carcinogenicity of organic compounds.

To improve the statistical certainty of our analysis, we have also made use of an additional source of information: the results of various *in vitro* experiments. Thus the analysis of the correlation between the AQVN and the carcinogenic activity of organic compounds attempted here involves approximately 600 different chemical agents. Because analytical results depend upon the type of experiment used, we will refer mainly to the Lyon data further on in this presentation, however.

The choice of IARC data did not, however, fully resolve all our practical problems. An important issue remained open: what criteria should be used to define the carcinogenicity of a particular substance? At first glance the application of those used by the IARC might seem the logical choice. But the question is not so easily answered because the IARC criteria take into account practical and commercial considerations for each given substance. It is more controversial to pronounce a widely-used substance as "carcinogenic", especially if there is no adequate substitute for it, than it is upon a substance with limited use, particularly if it can be satisfactorily replaced.

Since the effects of these practical judgemental considerations could not be eliminated, we opted for a compromise. Our analysis will be presented in two ways: in our first analysis we will consider as carcinogenic only those substances which are active by IARC criteria[2a] (compounds marked with an asterisk in Table 3), while in our second we will consider as carcinogenic all compounds that have been found to induce a significant number of malignant tumours in experiments *in vivo*.

Table 3 and Figure 4 show the AQVN and other data concerning the carcinogenicity of 316 organic compounds grouped according to their chemical type and in the order in which they are presented in IARC monographs. The histogram shows that the largest number of carcinogenic compounds lies in the AQVN range between 2.4 and 3.1. A lesser number of carcinogenic compounds occurs in the range below 2.4. Therefore the 2.4 value should be taken as a lower borderline separating the carcinogenic from the noncarcinogenic range.

The situation in the AQVN range above 3.1 is similar. There are many compounds in nature with AQVN's in this range (compounds with unsaturated chemical bonds, ones rich in oxygen, sulphur, nitrogen and phosphorus, a large family of heterocyclic compounds). It is not easy to evaluate the relative number of these compounds in nature. An analysis of samples covering several thousand compounds from different sources[21,22] shows AQVN values evenly distributed in the range between 2.0 and 3.9. In this way, $Z^* = 3.1$ constitutes the upper limit between potentially carcinogenic and noncarcinogenic agents. Of 287 carcinogenic compounds listed in Table 3, we see that 37 (*i.e.* 12.9%) have an AQVN of higher than 3.1. If only the compounds which are carcinogenic by IARC criteria[2a] (marked by asterisk in Table 3) are taken into account, the result changes slightly: out of a total of 121, 24 (*i.e.* 19.8%) fall in the AQVN range above 3.1.

If we observe the number of carcinogens in the unit AQVN-interval with a width of 0.10, we see that it is 5.14 times greater in the area between 2.4 and 3.1 than outside this area. For the carcinogens by IARC criteria[2a] this factor is 3.89, and 5.1 for definitive human carcinogens[2a]. This clearly confirms the applicability of the criterion.

These results may be used as a basis for a preselection test to determine the potential carcinogenicity of organic compounds: if a given chemical compound's AQVN-value falls in the area between 2.4 and 3.1, the probability that it is carcinogenic is 4–5 times greater than it would be if its AQVN-value were not in this area.

It may be observed that some of the above results (borderline values and percentages of carcinogens) differ to some extent from those presented in Ref. 23. This is a result of better data and a more stringent analysis of biological findings. One of the disadvantages of this analysis is connected with the relatively small number of noncarcinogenic agents tested. But there is an objective reason for this. The IARC monographs, as well as other sources, deal with compounds for which there are indications of carcinogenicity. Due to the high cost, the time needed and the complexity of experimental testing, research has concentrated much more on carcinogenic than on noncarcinogenic agents. But even the limited number of carcinogenic agents established by the IARC (see Table 3) has an AQVN distribution supporting the above conclusions. Of all these compounds, approximately 50% are in the range below and another 50% in the range above the 3.1 limit. Since these compounds were analysed together with carcinogens without any preliminary selection, this distribution points to the fact that noncarcinogenic agents are not characterized by any special grouping with respect to their AQVN's. This raises the logical possibility of there being some additional criterion which might allow us to separate carcinogenic from noncarcinogenic agents in the AQVN region between 2.4 and 3.1. A physical criterion of this kind will be considered in chapter 5.

Let us now consider two principal advantages which might be brought about by the use of such a correlation. First, this simple criterion might be used for the preliminary selection of potentially dangerous agents from the large set of commercially used chemicals, all of which must at some point be subjected to the protracted, complex and expensive biological testing procedure. A quicker, cheaper and more accurate way of determining those materials that are carcinogenic would thus be provided. Secondly, and this in our opinion is of primary importance, the correlation established between this physical parameter and carcinogenicity offers a new approach to the investigation of the mechanism of the complex biological phenomenon of chemical carcinogenesis. A large portion of the remainder of this presentation will concern itself with this issue in an attempt to discover the connection between the AQVN and essential biological properties which might be grounds for the established correlation.

Looking into some possible pitfalls in this approach, there is first the question of structural isomerism. We are all familiar with the experimentally confirmed role which this physical property plays in chemical carcinogenesis. Some structural isomers may show substantially different carcinogenic activity to others; nevertheless the effect of structural isomerism is not taken into account in determining the AQVN. At the same time, however, we have demonstrated a correlation between the AQVN and the carcinogenicity of organic compounds. This apparent contradiction can be explained in the following way: the AQVN constitutes a necessary but not a sufficient parameter as a measure of the carcinogenicity of organic compounds. The structural factor is an additional parameter.

Another matter pertaining to the correlation which may be confusing to the biologist or biochemist is the fact that this correlation has been determined without considering *in vivo* metabolic transformations of substances after entry into the human organism. This point deserves more attention. In most cases chemical compounds absorbed by the human body with the ingestion of foodstuffs and medications, or through the skin or respiratory process, undergo a series of gradual chemical transformations once they are inside. For this reason, at the end of the metabolic process we are no longer dealing with the original substance but with its metabolites, which, from the standpoint of biochemical activity, may substantially differ from the original substance. Therefore, we may rightfully ask why we should correlate a physicochemical characteristic of an organic agent with its carcinogenic effect if this is due to the agent's metabolites, which need not be chemically very similar to the original substance.

To explain the viability of the correlation between the AQVN and carcinogenicity with this question in mind, we should be familiar with the following:

1) The mechanism whereby a chemical carcinogen leads to the cancerization of the cell.

2) A sufficient number of metabolic pathways of individual carcinogens, so

TABLE 4

Changes of AQVN for some organic carcinogens caused by some metabolic processes.[2,43]

Substance	Z^*	ΔZ^*, %
Propham	2.69	
Metabolites:		
$C_{10}H_{13}NO_4$	2.93	8.92
$C_{10}H_{13}NO_3$	2.81	4.46
C_6H_7N	2.57	4.46
$C_8H_9NO_2$	2.90	7.81
Chloropropham	2.69	
Metabolites:		
$C_{10}H_{12}ClNO_3$	2.81	4.46
$C_{10}H_{12}ClNO_4$	2.93	8.92
C_6H_6ClN	2.57	4.46
C_6H_6ClNO	2.80	4.00
$C_8H_8ClNO_2$	2.90	7.81
$C_{10}H_{10}NO_4$	3.08	14.40
Benzopyrene	2.88	
Metabolites:		
$C_{20}H_{10}O$	3.10	7.64
$C_{20}H_{12}O_2$	3.06	6.25
$C_{20}H_{10}O_2$	3.10	10.76
$C_{21}H_{14}O$	2.89	0.35
Benzanthracene	2.80	
Metabolites:		
$C_{18}H_{12}O$	2.90	3.57
$C_{18}H_{14}O_2$	2.88	2.86

that we may draw some general conclusions about conditions under which metabolites take action.

Without these considerations the above question cannot be fully answered. For this reason we will analyse some metabolic pathways from the point of view of the AQVN.

Table 4 shows the AQVN's of some well-investigated chemical carcinogens and their metabolites.[2] This data points to the interesting fact that the difference between the AQVN of any metabolite and its initial substance does not exceed 10%. If we assume that other metabolic processes are in keeping with this 10% change then this explains how it was possible to establish the correlation between the AQVN and the carcinogenicity of organic agents without taking into account possible metabolic modifications to ultimate carcinogens.

If compounds are well within the range of potential carcinogens, having AQVN's far from the borderlines, or if they are well within the range of noncarcinogens (*i.e.* their AQVN's exceed 3.1 by a large margin), then their metabolites remain in the same AQVN range so that they do not alter their nature with respect to carcinogenicity. However, if a compound has an AQVN value near the 3.1 limit (plus or minus 0.3) the situation is different. Due to metabolic processes these compounds can change their original activity, since the AQVN's of their metabolites need not necessarily be in the same AQVN range as the initial substances.

If we examine the compounds listed in Table 3 which deviate from the observed correlation we find that the AQVN of almost all of them is in the 3.1 area, plus or minus 0.3. There are some exceptions but this is not surprising because the borderline between potential carcinogens and noncarcinogens was not established as a result of some physical or chemical criterion but as a result of experimental data. Hence, some agents may have metabolites of a very different activity or may be unstable compounds which undergo radical chemical change in the organism and divide into fragments with considerably modified AQVN's.

Finally, let us examine another important issue concerning the correlation between AQVN and cancer. In all experiments that suggest carcinogenic activity the question of whether we are justified in assuming that similar activity takes place in the human organism remains unanswered. To be more precise, are there any metabolic processes in the human organism that are capable of activating a substance which in other life forms manifests no carcinogenic properties? And, conversely, can metabolic processes in the human organism deactivate agents that produce cancer in other biological systems? It is because of these unanswered questions that it is extremely difficult to determine to what extent such experimental tests apply to man. At present, however, we have no better choice, and for this reason the tests are taken as valid on the grounds of probability.

The relationship between the correlation and metabolic transformations allows for an interesting hypothesis. On one hand the correlation is defined on the basis of experimental data regarding the carcinogenicity of organic agents obtained through the study of effects they induce in other mammalian systems; on the other hand it has been demonstrated that metabolic processes seldom change the AQVN of the initial substance by more than 10%. Several standard metabolic transformations taking place in the human organism are shown in Table 5. An analysis of these transformations leads to the conclusion that the correlation is also valid when dealing with the effect of organic agents in the human organism.

The AQVN borderline separating the regions of noncarcinogenic from potentially carcinogenic agents has not yet been considered from a biological, chemical or physical standpoint. We will nonetheless demonstrate that it may be related to some interesting biochemical and physicochemical characteristics.

TABLE 5

Analysis of normal metabolic processes from the aspect of average quasi-valence numbers.

Name	Formula	Z*	ΔZ*, %
Lysine	$C_6H_{14}N_2O_2$	2.50	
Keto-amino caproic acid	$C_6H_{11}NO_3$	2.76	10.4
Piperidine-2-carboxylic acid	$C_6H_9NO_2$	2.78	11.1
Pipecoloic acid	$C_6H_{10}NO_2$	2.68	7.2
Piperidine-6-carboxylic acid	$C_6H_9NO_2$	2.78	11.1
Aminoadipic acid semialdehyde	$C_6H_{11}NO_3$	2.76	10.4
Colamine	C_2H_7NO	2.36	
Methylaminoethanol	C_3H_9NO	2.71	15.0
Dimethylaminoethanol	$C_4H_{10}NO$	2.31	2.1
Choline	$C_5H_{15}NO_2$	2.26	4.4
Tyrosine	$C_9H_{11}NO_3$	2.92	
Dioxyphenylalanine	$C_9H_{11}NO_4$	3.04	4.1
Dopamine	$C_8H_{11}NO_2$	2.73	6.8
Noradrenaline	$C_8H_{11}NO_2$	2.73	6.5
Adrenaline	$C_9H_{13}NO_3$	2.77	5.1

Let us examine the distribution of the main components of living matter, amino acids and purine and pyrimidine bases, with respect to their AQVN's. Determining the AQVN's of these molecules gives rise to the following question: would it be more appropriate to consider the AQVN of a free molecule or of a molecule built into a protein chain, DNA or RNA? Tables 6 and 7 and Figure 5 give the corresponding AQVN values for both forms; for a free molecule and for an active molecular group. In our subsequent analysis we will use AQVN's of the active molecular groups.

Figure 6 shows that the borderline between the AQVN of amino acids on one hand and purine and pyrimidine bases on the other is approximately 3.1. The range of amino acids fully overlaps with the range of potential chemical carcinogens. An interesting hypothesis derived from this fact is that chemical carcinogens may act in living matter in some connection with amino acids. Some experimental facts which we shall later examine indicate to us that this possibility is not unlikely.

Experimental data concerning the activity of organic carcinogens demonstrate that each carcinogen usually causes one type or a specific group of tumours, independent of the system it is affecting. In the course of a broader analysis of the carcinogenicity of organic agents, from the point of view of the AQVN, we also examined the distribution of the AQVN for agents causing the most frequent types of cancer. Table 3 provides data for carcinogens causing hepatoma, adenocarcinoma, papilloma and sarcoma. Figure 7 presents the relative distribution of the AQVN of agents causing each of these tumours

TABLE 6
Average quasi-valence numbers (Z^*) of amino acids, purine and pyrimidine bases and nucleic acid derivatives.

Substance	Formula	Z^*
Amino acids		
Leucine (+)	$C_6H_{13}NO_2$	2.45
Isoleucine (+)	$C_6H_{13}NO_2$	2.45
Lysine (+)	$C_6H_{14}N_2O_2$	2.50
Valine (+)	$C_5H_{11}NO_2$	2.53
Threonine (+)	$C_4H_9NO_2$	2.63
Arginine (+)	$C_6H_{14}N_4O_2$	2.69
Proline	$C_5H_9NO_2$	2.71
Alanine	$C_3H_7NO_2$	2.77
Phenylalanine (+)	$C_9H_{11}NO_2$	2.78
Asparagine	$C_4H_8N_2O_2$	2.88
Methionine (+)	$C_5H_9NO_2S$	2.89
Tryptophan (+)	$C_{11}H_{12}N_2O_2$	2.89
Glutamine	$C_5H_{10}N_2O_3$	2.90
Tyrosine	$C_9H_{11}NO_3$	2.92
Histidine (+)	$C_6H_9N_3O_2$	3.00
Serine	$C_3H_7NO_3$	3.00
Glycine	$C_2H_5NO_3$	3.00
Cysteine	$C_3H_7NO_2S$	3.00
Glutamate	$C_5H_8N_2O_3$	3.11
Aspartate	$C_4H_7NO_4$	3.25
Purine and pyrimidine base		
Thymine	$C_5H_6N_2O_2$	3.20
Cytosine	$C_4H_5N_3O$	3.23
Adenine	$C_5H_5N_5$	3.33
Guanine	$C_5H_5N_5O$	3.50
Uracil	$C_4H_4N_2O_2$	3.50
Nucleic acid derivatives		
Purines:		
2-Aminopurine	$C_5H_5N_5$	3.33
2,6-Diaminopurine	$C_5H_6N_6$	3.29
2,8-Dioxyadenine	$C_5H_5N_5O_2$	3.65
Hypoxanthine	$C_5H_4N_4O$	3.57
Isoguanine	$C_5H_5N_5O$	3.50
Purine	$C_5H_4N_4$	3.38
Uric acid	$C_5H_4N_4O_3$	3.88
Xanthine	$C_5H_4N_4O_2$	3.73
Pyrimidines:		
5-Hydroxymethylcytosine	$C_5H_7N_3O_2$	3.18
5-Methylcytosine	$C_5H_7N_3O$	3.00
Orotic acid	$C_5H_4N_2O$	3.87
Ribonucleosides:		
Adenosine	$C_{10}H_{13}N_5O_4$	3.19
Cytidine	$C_9H_{13}N_3O_5$	3.13
2,6-Diaminopurine ribonucleoside	$C_{10}H_{14}N_6O_4$	3.18
Guanosine	$C_{10}H_{13}N_5O_5$	3.27
Inosine	$C_{10}H_{12}N_4O_5$	3.29
Isoguanine ribonucleoside	$C_{10}H_{13}N_5O_5$	3.27

Substance	Formula	Z^*
Orotidine	$C_{10}H_{12}N_2O_8$	3.44
Pseudouridine	$C_9H_{12}N_2O_6$	3.24
Purine ribonucleoside	$C_{10}H_{12}N_4O_4$	3.20
5-Methylcytidine	$C_{10}H_{15}N_3O_5$	3.03
Uric acid ribonucleoside	$C_{10}H_{12}N_4O_7$	3.45
Uridine	$C_9H_{12}N_2O_6$	3.24
Xanthosine	$C_{10}H_{12}N_4O_6$	3.38
2'-Deoxyribonucleosides:		
Deoxyadenosine	$C_{10}H_{13}N_5O_3$	3.10
Deoxycytidine	$C_9H_{13}N_3O_4$	3.03
Deoxyguanosine	$C_{10}H_{13}N_5O_4$	3.19
Deoxyinosine	$C_{10}H_{12}N_4O_4$	3.20
5-Methyldeoxycytidine	$C_{10}H_{15}N_3O_4$	2.94
Thymidine	$C_{10}H_{14}N_2O_5$	3.03
Deoxyuridine	$C_9H_{12}N_2O_5$	3.14
Deoxyxanthosine	$C_{10}H_{12}N_4O_5$	3.29
5'-Deoxyribonucleotides:		
Deoxyadenylic acid	$C_{10}H_{14}N_5O_6P$	3.33
Deoxycytidilic acid	$C_9H_{14}N_3O_7P$	3.29
Deoxyguanylic acid	$C_{10}H_{14}N_5O_7P$	3.40
Deoxy-5-methylcytidylic acid	$C_{10}H_{16}N_3O_7P$	3.19
Thymidilic acid	$C_{10}H_{15}N_2O_8P$	3.28
Deoxyribonucleoside diphosphates:		
Deoxycytidine-3,5'-diphosphate	$C_9H_{15}N_3O_{10}P_2$	3.49
Thymidine-3'-diphosphate	$C_{10}H_{16}N_2O_{11}P_2$	3.46

(+)   Essential amino acids.

individually, as well as the relative distribution of all the carcinogens analysed and the twenty basic amino acids.

It is noteworthy that the largest number of agents causing all four types of carcinomas lie in the AQVN range 2.6–3.0. Tyrosine, tryptophan, histidine, glutamine, glutamic acid and asparagine are all within these limits. This reopens the question of the role of amino acids in cell cancerization. In view of the available data and relevant statistics it is difficult to believe that this overlapping of AQVN's is purely coincidental.

Another interesting conclusion may be derived from Figure 7. The largest number of carcinogenic agents causing the most frequent carcinomas (mentioned above) fall in the AQVN range between 2.8 and 2.9. This is indicative of the intensified activity of agents in this particular region, and should certainly be taken into account in the preselection of organic compounds for purposes of both testing and application.

On the other hand, the situation is completely different with chemical agents causing neurocarcinomas. Table 8 offers a survey of these agents, showing that the AQVN's of agents inducing neurocarcinoma overlap with the AQVN's of

TABLE 7

Active groups of amino acids and their quasi-valence numbers.

Name	Abbreviation	R	Z^*
Glycine	gly	$-H$	1.00
Alanine	ala	$-CH_3$	1.75
Valine	val	$-CH\overset{CH_3}{\underset{CH_3}{}}$	1.90
Leucine	leu	$-CH_2-CH\overset{CH_3}{\underset{CH_3}{}}$	1.92
Isoleucine	ile	$-CH-CH_2-CH_3$ $\quad\ \ \vert$ $\quad\ CH_3$	1.92
Proline	pro	$-CH_2\quad CH_2$ $\quad\ \ \underset{CH_2}{\diagdown}$	2.00
Lysine	lys	$-CH_2-CH_2-CH_2-CH_2-NH_2$	2.07
Methionine	met	$-CH_2-CH_2-S-CH_3$	2.27
Threonine	thr	$-CH\overset{OH}{\underset{CH_3}{}}$	2.38
Arginine	arg	$-CH_2-CH_2-CH_2-NH-C\overset{NH_2}{\underset{NH}{}}$	2.41
Phenylalanine	phe	$-CH_2-\hexagon$	2.50
Serine	der	$-CH_2-OH$	2.60
Cysteine	cys	$-CH_2-SH$	2.60
Glutamine	glu	$-CH_2-CH_2-CONH_2$	2.64
Tryptophan	try	$-CH_2-$ (indole ring)	2.72
Tyrosine	tyr	$-CH_2-\hexagon-OH$	2.73
Histidine	his	$-CH_2-$ (imidazole ring)	2.82
Asparagine	asn	$-CH_2-CONH_2$	2.88
Glutamic acid	glu	$-CH_2-CH_2-COOH$	2.90
Aspartic acid	asp	$-CH_2-COOH$	3.29

purine and pyrimidine bases. This distinguishes them radically from other chemical carcinogens causing the types of tumours already mentioned and indicates that chemical carcinogens may affect nerve tissue in a different way. In view of the particular nature of nerve cells (*i.e.* these cells are not subject to division), this should not come as any surprise.

The chemotherapy of neurocarcinoma points in the same direction. Figure 11 clearly shows that alkylating cytostatics, which act effectively in the majority of cancer diseases, are within the AQVN region of amino acids. If the

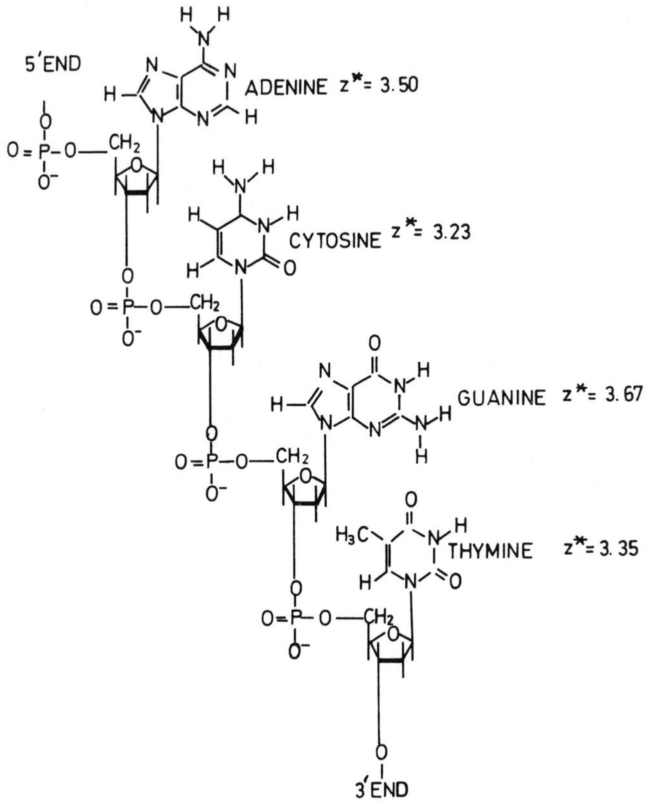

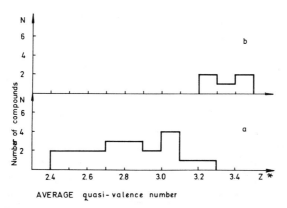

FIGURE 5   Effective average quasi-valence numbers of nucleotides in the structure of DNA.

FIGURE 6   Distribution, with respect to their average quasi-valence numbers, of a) amino acids
and b) nucleotides.

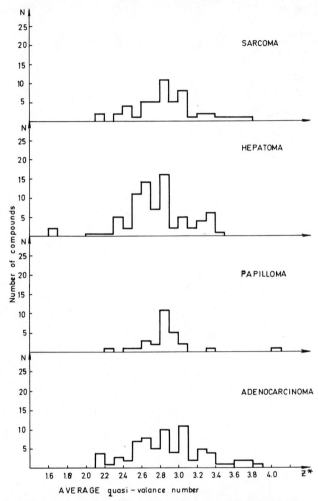

FIGURE 7   Distribution, with respect to their average quasi-valence numbers, of the agents known to cause some of the more frequent forms of tumours.

former hypothesis is true, *i.e.* if the cancerization of nerve tissue is not related in some way to amino acids, then alkylating cytostatics should not be expected to have a therapeutic effect in the case of neurocarcinoma. Clinical practice fully confirms this finding.[24] Unlike alkylating agents, antimetabolic cytostatics, whose AQVN's overlap with the AQVN's of purines and pyrimidines, should have a therapeutic effect on these tumours, and this too has been confirmed in clinical practice.[24]

It should be pointed out here that our analysis involved only those chemical

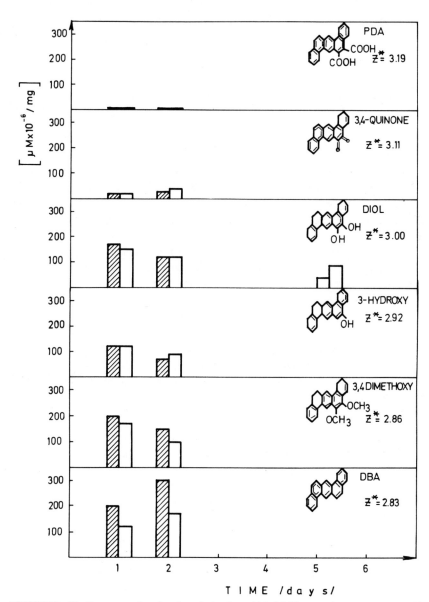

FIGURE 8 Binding properties of various derivatives of 1,2,5,6-dibenzanthracene to mouse-skin proteins. Specific activity (micromoles $\times 10^{-6}$ equivalents per milligram of dried protein) against time in days. Solid bars represent soluble proteins; open bars represent particulates.

TABLE 8

Average quasi-valence number Z^* of some neurocarcinogens.

Substance	Chemical formula	Z^*
Nitrosomethylurea	$C_2H_5N_3O_2$	3.33
Nitrosoethylurea	$C_3H_7N_3O_2$	3.07
1,3-Propane sultone	$C_3H_6O_3S$	3.23
Dimethyl sulphate	$C_2H_6O_4S$	3.38
Methyl methanesulphonate	$C_2H_6O_3S$	3.17

carcinogens about which we could obtain data demonstrating the results of their oral administration into mammalian systems. This selection was made in order to provide similar conditions of metabolic transformations for all compounds analysed. This requirement was not applied to agents causing neurocarcinoma, since to date only a few of them have been described in the literature.

There are other experimental data obtained for proteins which also point to the crucial role of amino acids in chemical carcinogenesis. One experiment, for example, has demonstrated that the carcinogenicity of 1,2,5,6-dibenzanthracene and its derivatives is directly proportional to the extent to which these agents bind themselves to the proteins in the skin of mice.[25] What is even more interesting is the fact that from the standpoint of the AQVN's of these compounds, the binding of agents to proteins ceases as their AQVN's approach the 3.1 borderline (see Figure 8). This is yet another indication that the correlation between the AQVN's of chemical carcinogens and amino acids is no coincidence.

Finally, let us summarize the conclusions drawn in this chapter.

1) There is a correlation between the carcinogenic activity of organic compounds and their AQVN's, and this correlation may be used in a preliminary selection of potentially carcinogenic agents.

2) The overlapping of AQVN's of organic carcinogens and amino acids is indicative of the possible role of amino acids in the process of chemical carcinogenesis.

These findings demonstrate that the AQVN is a suitable physical parameter which may be useful in the study of chemical carcinogenesis.

CHAPTER 4

The Role of the Average Quasi-Valence Number in Biological Systems

The results of the previous analysis give rise to the important question of on what physical basis this simple parameter, the AQVN, correlates with a biological phenomenon as complex as chemical carginogenesis. For a number of reasons it is practically impossible fully to answer this question. First, we do not sufficiently understand certain processes taking place in living matter, especially those related to the chemical cancerization of a cell. Secondly, current theoretical knowledge does not allow us to study these complex phenomena from the perspective of elementary interactions. This situation unfortunately exists in the majority of vital biological processes, notwithstanding advancements made in the fields of molecular biology, genetics, biochemistry and biophysics.

To arrive at some physical explanation for the correlation between the AQVN and chemical carcinogenicity in spite of the above-mentioned difficulties, we resorted to the phenomenological approach, it being the only available choice in a situation where theory has not yet reached a level of development to permit a more exact method of handling the problem. Practice has shown that such an approach may be useful, since insights thus obtained may often be of great importance in the development of new theory.

To learn more about the role of the AQVN in biological processes, a number of characteristics of living matter were examined with this physical parameter in mind. At the end of this chapter we will draw a phenomenological sketch of the role of the AQVN in biological systems, paying special attention to the phenomenon of chemical carcinogenesis.

Now we will analyse the hydrophilic properties of chemical compounds with respect to the AQVN. We chose this physicochemical property because it plays such an important role in biological processes. As we know, this phenomenon manifests itself in the grouping of water dipoles around an ion or polar molecule present in a solution. The width of this hydration layer depends upon the strength of the interaction between water dipoles and ions or molecules. Since all biological processes occur in a water medium, the process of hydration is of great importance. The hydration layer around molecules participating in biological processes is defined by its effective diameter. The effective diameter of a molecule in turn substantially affects the dynamics of its

TABLE 9
Hydrophilic and hydrophobic groups and their AQVN (Z^*).

Hydrophilic groups	Z^*	Hydrophobic group	Z^*
–SH	3.50	$-C_3H_7$	1.90
–O–	6.00	$-C_2H_5$	1.86
$-C\overset{O}{\underset{OH}{\diagup}}$	4.25	$-CH_3$	1.75
$-C\overset{O}{\underset{NH_2}{\diagup}}$	3.40	$-CH=CH_2$	2.20
$-\underset{\overset{\|}{O}}{C}-$	5.50	$-CCl_3$	1.75
–OH	3.50	$-CF_3$	1.75
$-\overset{O}{\underset{O}{\overset{\|}{\underset{\|}{S}}}}-OH$	5.00	⬡—	2.63
H_2O	2.67		
$-C\overset{O}{\underset{H}{\diagup}}$	3.67		

transportation through a biological system. This effect is highly enhanced when molecules are passing through membrane systems in tissue.

The binding of water to organic molecules is due to interaction between the positive pole of the water molecule dipole and the cloud of electrons belonging to the organic molecule. The stronger the interaction the larger the number of water molecules in the hydration layer and, consequently, the larger its effective diameter. The density of the negative molecular charge, which largely determines the strength of the interaction, is roughly proportional to the value of the AQVN of this molecule. Thus the AQVN is an indirect indication of the hydration properties of organic molecules.

Following the same principle, we know that water molecules establish hydrogen bonds between themselves. In order to bind a water dipole, *i.e.* to be hydrophilic, an organic molecule must interact with the water dipole more strongly than the water molecules interact with each other. From the point of view of charge this means that the AQVN of any given molecule must exceed that of water. This is by no means the only condition which must be met in the case of a hydrophilic molecule, but it is the main one. Several examples will be given to demonstrate the importance of the AQVN as a criterion for hydrophilicity.

Table 9 contains data on the AQVN and hydrophilicity of some markedly hydrophilic and hydrophobic groups.[26] As we can see from this data, the

TABLE 10

Vitamins and their quasi-valence numbers.

Vitamin	Formula	Z^*
Vitamins soluble in water		
B_1 (Thiamine)	$C_{12}H_{17}N_4OSCl$	2.88
B_2 (Riboflavin)	$C_{17}H_{20}N_4O_6$	3.06
B_6 (Pyridoxine)	$C_8H_{11}NO_3$	2.87
B_{12} (Cyanocobalamin)	$C_{61}H_{86}N_{14}O_{13}PCo$	2.79
H (Biotin)	$C_{10}H_{16}N_2SO_3$	2.81
PP	$C_6H_6N_2O$	3.07
Inositol	$C_6H_{12}O_6$	3.00
Pantothenic acid	$C_9H_{17}NO_5$	2.75
para-Aminobenzoic acid	$C_7H_7NO_2$	3.06
Folic acid	$C_{19}H_{19}N_7O_6$	3.25
C (Ascorbic acid)	$C_6H_8O_6$	3.40
Vitamins soluble in fats		
A (Axerophtol)	$C_{20}H_{30}O$	2.27
D_2 (Calciferol)	$C_{28}H_{44}O$	2.22
D_3	$C_{27}H_{44}O$	2.19
D_4	$C_{28}H_{46}O$	2.19
E (Tocopherol)	$C_{29}H_{50}O_2$	2.20
K_1 (3-Phytylmenadione)	$C_{31}H_{46}O_2$	2.30
K_2 (3-Difarnesylmenadione)	$C_{41}H_{56}O_2$	2.04
F (Linoleic acid)	$C_{18}H_{32}O_2$	2.11

AQVN's of all hydrophilic groups are higher than the AQVN of water, which is 2.67. At the same time, the AQVN's of all hydrophobic groups fall below this value.

Now let us take a look at vitamins, those vital participants in a great number of biochemical processes occurring in the human organism. They are divided into two groups; vitamins soluble in water and those soluble in fats. The AQVN values for both groups are presented in Table 10. We can see that the water-soluble variety must be of a hydrophilic nature.

It is noteworthy that both these groups of vitamins are grouped around two AQVN values, with surprisingly small mean deviations from these respective values. Water-soluble vitamins are grouped around $Z^* = 2.92$, with a mean deviation of 3.8%, while the fat soluble ones are grouped around $Z^* = 2.19$, with a mean deviation of 2.7%. This fact is quite interesting when we bear in mind that fats found in the human organism are grouped around $Z^* = 2.20$, with a mean deviation of 1.8%. It is difficult to imagine that such a highly specific AQVN grouping as that of vitamins does not possess some biological importance. For now we wish to call attention to the fact that the number of atoms per molecule of vitamin varies considerably, ranging from 22 to 176, and that these vitamins belong to different chemical types.

Now let us examine the amino acids from the perspective of hydrophilic characteristics. The biological amino acids all have the universal form

NH_2–CHR–COOH, which by polycondensation forms the basic protein structure. We will dwell at some length on the active side components, R, of the amino acids, since these define their principal nature, while the universal backbone remnant constitutes a constant. Table 7 presents the AQVN's of the 20 active groups of the basic biological amino acids. The mean value of the AQVN's of active amino acid groups is $Z^* = 2.36$.

The hydrophilicity of these functional groups plays a decisive role in the formation of higher (tertiary and quaternary) protein structures. These higher structures are important, being responsible for the proper functioning of proteins in any given biological system. Disruption or change of these higher configurations leads to the disruption or loss of the protein function. One characteristic example is the well-known disease sickle cell anaemia. In people affected by this disease normal haemoglobin is replaced by deformed haemoglobin, the so-called haemoglobin S. Glutamic acid in haemoglobin S is replaced by valine. The substitution of the hydrophilic component (glutamic acid) by a hydrophobic one (valine) so profoundly affects the configuration of the haemoglobin molecule that it loses its oxygen-carrying ability.

The grouping, according to effective AQVN's, of the amino acids with the most pronounced hydrophilic (or hydrophobic) characteristics[27] is in full accord with what might be expected as a result of previous findings. The effective AQVN's of hydrophilic amino acids are above 2.6, while those of the hydrophobic ones are below this value. If we exclude cysteine, which is at the borderline between the hydrophilic and hydrophobic regions, we find that of all amino acids presented, only arginine and lysine deviate from the above classification. This mismatch is most probably caused by the special chain-like structure of amino acids (see Table 7) resulting in a different activity of groups at the beginning and end of the chain in their interactions with other molecules. A study of this mismatch will no doubt contribute to the understanding of the physical background of the correlation between hydrophilicity and the AQVN.

These findings provide a basic idea about the physicochemical grounds for the role played by the AQVN in biological systems. In the case of chemical carcinogens, the effective diameter of their molecules probably constitutes one of the more important parameters affecting their activity. From this point of view, the correlation between the AQVN and carcinogenicity acquires some of its physical significance.

On the other hand, the average quasi-valence number in some respect represents the average electron density in the electron cloud belonging to a given molecule. Noncarcinogens, that is organic molecules which have high AQVN's (> 3.1), behave like agents with nucleophilic (electron-rich) centres. Potential carcinogens have smaller AQVN's (in the range 2.4–3.1) and therefore a lower electron cloud density. They act as agents characterized by the possession of electrophilic (electron deficient) centres. According to a modern theory of chemical carcinogenesis the existence of electrophilic centres in rather simple organic molecules coupled with the existence of nucleophilic centres in macromolecules (proteins, RNA and DNA) is responsible for the initiation of the complex phenomenon which leads to the cancerization of the cell caused by the action of chemical carcinogens.[26]

According to Prof. A. Szent-Gyorgyi, a possible explanation for different biochemical activities of organic compounds having low or high AQVN's might be sought in their acceptor-like or donor-like behaviour.[28]

The analysis which follows will give some indication of the behaviour of complete protein macromolecules with respect to the effective AQVN. We will inquire as to what might be expected, in view of the available information on amino acids.

The mean effective AQVN value of the 20 basic amino acids listed in Table 7 is 2.36. This same table demonstrates that the effective AQVN's of twelve of the amino acids are above this value. From a statistical point of view we might therefore expect the mean effective AQVN for all amino acids of a macro-molecule to be higher than, or equal to, this value. Furthermore, we should expect this to be true for all proteins, since so far no protein has been found that has a markedly higher content of any particular amino acid (with the exception of a certain class of histones rich in arginine and lysine). Expecta-tions aside, let us now look at the actual situation.

Table 11 presents the composition of several of the approximately 70 analysed proteins, containing over 6000 amino acids and originating in different biological systems, ranging from viruses to man. All of these analysed proteins were grouped around an effective AQVN value of 2.25, with a mean deviation of 3%. At first glance this deviation from the anticipated mean value of 2.36 might seem negligible; nonetheless, if we bear in mind that these proteins are made up of combinations of only 20 amino acids with no specific protein preference, then this discrepancy is significant. Only histones deviate from this rule, but they have the special function of controlling genetic information. They are grouped around an effective AQVN value of 2.14, with a mean deviation of 2.9%. Some examples are presented in Table 12.

It is interesting to note how this characteristic affects shorter protein segments. We observed the same tendency in segments composed of not more than ten or fifteen amino acids. This interesting characteristic, observed in a large number of different proteins, will be illustrated by the example of histone from the thymus of the calf.[29] We considered the primary structure and effective AQVN of this protein for each segment surrounding DNA. All of these segments have extremely similar effective AQVN values, being grouped around 2.22, with a mean deviation of 2.6%. Statistically speaking, this regularity governing short protein segments is more surprising than it is in

TABLE 11
Proteins and their AQVN (Z^*).

Protein	Biological system	Number of amino acids	Z^*	Ref.
A-protein	Bacteriophage MS2	533	2.23	(41)
Growth hormone	Rat	215	2.27	(42)
Ribosomal protein				(61)
S4	E. coli	203	2.25	
S15	E. coli	87	2.28	
S21	E. coli	70	2.27	
L25	E. coli	94	2.23	
L27	E. coli	63	2.27	
L32	E. coli	56	2.25	
L29	E. coli	63	2.27	
L33	E. coli	54	2.21	
β-Globin	Rabbit	146	2.22	(62)
Insulin	Bovine	52	2.29	(27)
Lysozyme	Human	129	2.29	(63)
β-Haemoglobin	Human	146	2.19	(63)
Rp2-L	Walker 256 carcinosarcoma	—	1.97	(30)

TABLE 12
Histones of calf thymus[29] and their AQVN (Z^*).

Histone	Number of amino acids	Z^*
F2b	125	2.19
F2a1	102	2.06
F2a2	129	2.10
F3	135	2.19
F1	73	2.01

complete protein macromolecules with 200 or more components.

The analysis of proteins from the perspective of the effective AQVN is indicative of the fact that they are not statistical by-products of amino acids, but rather that the relationships between their components follow certain rules which are more or less the same for all proteins. In view of the diversity of systems to which they may be applied, the origin of these relationships might probably be found in the evolution of living matter.

It may be assumed that the binding of hydrophobic amino acids observed in this study has its functional significance. If we take note of the fact that the majority of proteins found in malignant cells have relatively low effective

AQVN values (around 2.0) which are within and below the histone range (see the example of the Rp2-L protein from Walker's 256 carcinosarcoma,[30] and see Table 11), it becomes clear that this distribution of amino acids in proteins also affects the phenomenon of carcinogenesis.

All these diverse findings are indicative of a connection between the AQVN, some characteristics of biological systems, and processes in living matter. They confirm that the correlation between the average quasi-valence number and chemical carcinogenicity has an important biophysical significance. We believe that a study contributing to the comprehension of these findings would no doubt help in understanding the mechanism of chemical carcinogenesis.

CHAPTER 5

The Correlation Between the Carcinogenicity of Organic Substances and their Spectral Characteristics

As we have seen, the AQVN may serve as a criterion for the division of organic agents into potential carcinogens and noncarcinogens. After obtaining these results our next step was to find an additional criterion which could be used to distinguish carcinogenic from noncarcinogenic agents in the 2.4–3.1 AQVN range. This was no simple task, since we had no indication whatsoever as to which direction should be taken.

While considering the well-established fact that carcinomas can be induced by agents of a highly diversified nature, such as u.v. radiation, chemicals and oncogenic viruses, we came to the conclusion that it would be realistic to assume that oncogenic information (we might call it the "cancer DNA") might be present in the cell prior to the activity of the carcinogenic agent.[31] We further hypothesized that this "cancer DNA" is part of the normal cellular DNA but is inactive and firmly blocked in the cell.[32] This is consistent with another well-known fact that in differentiated cells of higher organisms a large portion of the DNA is non-functional. Some of the vital characteristics of malignant cells, such as the loss of contact inhibition, highly intensive metabolic processes, loss of specific functions, etc., demonstrate a certain similarity between these cells and primitive organisms. This, in turn, provides evidence for the possibility that the "cancer DNA" is present as a result of the evolutionary history of higher organisms and thus may be a sort of fingerprint of the initial stages of the evolutionary process. It is difficult to speculate whether this part of the DNA becomes overactivated during the development and life of an organism under normal conditions. Certain characteristics of embryonic tissue indicate the possibility that this part of the genetic information is used in the development of the embryo until the gastrula stage, at which time a large number of undifferentiated cells must develop relatively quickly. Further differentiation leads to the development of cells with precisely defined functions in the organism.

If we accept this hypothesis about the existence of blocked oncogenic information in every cell, then the most important step in carcinogenesis turns out to be the process of *unblocking the "cancer DNA"*. Since various cancer-

TABLE 13
Experimental determination of carcinogenic wavelengths.[33]

Wavelength, nm	Animal	Tumour induction
230	Rat	+
230	Mouse	+
254	Mouse	+
270	Rat	+
282	Mouse	+
320	Rat	−
334	Rat	−
334	Mouse	−
400	Rat	−
400	Mouse	−
411	Mouse	−

inducing agents produce identical results, we assume that the mechanism by which oncogenic information is released is not dependent upon the nature of any particular carcinogenic agent.

In order to gain an understanding of the problem of the unblocking of the "cancer DNA", we chose ultraviolet radiation as the simplest cancer-inducing agent. Radiation is a *purely physical agent*, characterized by only one parameter: *energy*. In the case of radiation, the unblocking of "cancer DNA" depends solely on the introduction of a specific energy. The range of wavelengths of cancer-inducing ultraviolet radiations varies between 233 and 278 nm (see Table 13 and Ref. 33).

The above assumptions and experimental findings on the carcinogenic activity of u.v. radiation prompted us to analyse the u.v. absorption spectra of chemical carcinogens. Data on the activity of u.v. radiation indicated that it might be possible to find in the absorption spectra of organic carcinogens the peak(s) in the wavelength range between 230–282 nm, or somewhere close to this interval. Findings of this u.v.-absorption spectra analysis are presented in Table 3 and Figure 9.

Out of 138 organic compounds contained in the IARC monographs (Vol. 1-16) for which u.v.-absorption spectra are quoted, 118 are carcinogenic, while 20 are noncarcinogenic agents. Of the 118 carcinogenic agents listed in Table 3, 72% have their absorption peak(s) in the wavelength region from 210–260 nm. We may conclude from this data that there is a correlation between u.v. spectral characteristics and the carcinogenic activity of organic compounds. The mean concentration of chemical carcinogens per one nanometer in the wavelength interval 210–260 nm is 1.7. Outside this interval, in the range 200–500 nm, the density of chemical carcinogens (number of carcinogens per nm) is 0.11. The ratio between these two "densities" is 15.3. This means that for compounds having u.v. absorption peak(s) in the range 210–260 nm, the

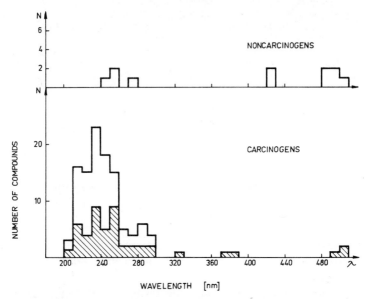

FIGURE 9 Relationship between carcinogenicity of chemical substances,[2] and their u.v.-spectral characteristics (carcinogens according IARC criteria are shaded).[2a]

probability of their being carcinogenic is 15.3 times higher than for compounds having no peak(s) in this spectral region. From this correlation we may conclude that compounds whose absorption spectral peak(s) are in the 210–286 nm range are most likely to be carcinogenic.

In this case, as in the case of the correlation between the AQVN and carcinogenicity, the borderline of the spectral range of carcinogens is empirical. This is probably one of the reasons why a certain number of carcinogenic agents deviate from the rule. In other words, approximately half of all carcinogenic agents for which deviation was observed are in the immediate proximity of the above-mentioned borderline values. The effect of solvents on the position of absorption peak(s) should not be disregarded either. In determining the u.v. spectra, mostly standard solvents were used;[34] even then there is a shift in absorption peak(s) of several nanometers, causing in the borderline region a deviation from the correlation found. The third and most important cause for deviation may be the metabolic process. The problem is, in fact, the same as that discussed in the case of the correlation between the AQVN and carcinogenicity. Unfortunately, in this particular case we could not carry out even a phenomenological study of the effects of metabolic processes on the change in spectral characteristics of organic carcinogens. The fact that the correlation between the u.v. spectra and the carcinogenic activity of organic compounds does indeed exist allows us only to assume that the situation is not drastically different from the one we met in the first correlation.

Figure 9 shows the distribution of noncarcinogenic agents presented in Table 3. It is important to note that noncarcinogenic agents do not group themselves around a certain narrow band of wavelengths. Most of the noncarcinogens are outside of the 210–260 nm interval.

The two correlations we have determined, that between spectral characteristics and the carcinogenic activity of organic compounds, and the one between the AQVN and the carcinogenicity of organic agents, may be combined to form one criterion: *organic compounds with an average quasi-valence number in the region between 2.4–3.1 and absorption peak(s) within the band of wavelengths ranging from 210–260 nm should be considered, with high probability, to be potential carcinogens.* Organic compounds which do not meet these conditions are most probably noncarcinogenic. As we have suggested, according to available data, the deviation from this rule totals 20.7 %. It should be recalled that this is the deviation from the most reliable biological experimental data available. These findings demonstrate that the above criterion may be very useful as an indication of the carcinogenicity of organic compounds and therefore may be useful as a preselection test.

Figure 10 shows the application of this criterion to IARC data (our Table 3). The AQVN interval 2.4–3.1 and wavelength range 210–260 nm taken together form an "island", covering the majority of carcinogenic agents. Findings presented in Table 3 indicate that some organic substances which cause certain types of cancer cover a broad range of wavelengths, as in the case of adenocarcinoma. Carcinogens inducing papilloma, for example, cover a narrower wavelength band.

Along with its usefulness as a criterion for the preselection of organic compounds according to their carcinogenicity, the correlation between u.v. absorption spectra and carcinogenicity offers some important insights into the mechanism of carcinogenesis. Owing to this correlation we are for the first time able to define the common characteristic responsible for the carcinogenic activity of two completely different agents: u.v. radiation and chemical carcinogens.

If carcinogenesis is analysed in the light of the data we have presented here, several hypotheses which may be valuable in understanding of the mechanism of this process may be distinguished. First we may assume that oncogenic information is present in the genetic information of every cell. Two essential facts support this assumption:

1) Approximately 200 types of malignant cells have so far been identified, each characterized by certain complex genetic information. Certainly this information cannot emanate from mutational changes in normal cellular information; if it did, the number of possibilities would be much larger. The

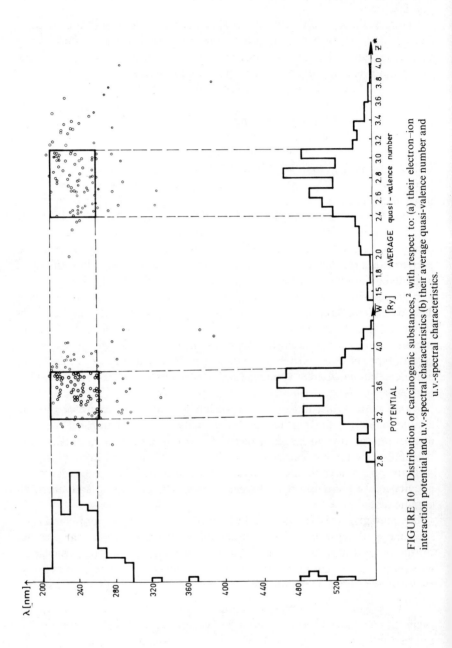

FIGURE 10   Distribution of carcinogenic substances,[2] with respect to: (a) their electron-ion interaction potential and u.v.-spectral characteristics (b) their average quasi-valence number and u.v.-spectral characteristics.

same applies to information introduced by oncogenic viruses: the information carried by viruses is not sufficient to "design" a complete malignant cell, which, in comparison with a virus, represents a much more complex system. Nor can it be assumed that the "cancer DNA" is a product of the combination of genetic information of several viruses. More than 100 oncogenic viruses are known today, the number of their possible combinations greatly exceeding the known number of malignant cell types. This fact does not allow us to hypothesize that the "cancer DNA" results from viral contamination of human DNA, but supports the assumption that it is the result of evolution.[32]

2) It is well known that any cellular culture grown *in vitro* under specific conditions (*e.g.* density of cells in the culture, pH, temperature) is subject to spontaneous cancerization, even though the cells are not exposed to the action of any carcinogenic agent.[35] This is possible only if the cells of a given culture already contain the "cancer DNA."

In the light of this analysis, if we accept the hypothesis that oncogenic information is present in every cell, then the process involved in its unblocking represents the most important step in cell cancerization. The data we have presented indicates that a particular energy might be held responsible for the initiation of cancer, although present-day knowledge unfortunately does not allow us to define the manner in which this energetic process takes place. We will not go into an analysis of possible hypothetical mechanisms, since there are too many of them. Instead, we will present some data which may prove useful in speculations of this sort.

First let us again make reference to the work of Szent-Gyorgyi, who established the correlation between the excitation level maximum of chemical carcinogens and the width of the energy gap between valence electrons and the conduction band of proteins.[36] As we found, the energies in the u.v. absorption spectra of organic carcinogens in the wavelength band from 210–260 nm are close to the width of the prohibited energy gap in the protein.[37] The experimentally established interaction between chemical carcinogens and the protein content of a cell should also be taken as supporting evidence.[38,39]

It is also important to mention the characteristics of steroid hormones. Their spectral characteristics and carcinogenicity are presented in Table 14. As this data indicates, all hormones listed are carcinogenic and their absorption peaks are within the range of other chemical carcinogens. It is also noteworthy that they play a major role in the cellular differentiation process, which ultimately means the unblocking of existing genetic information.

Something may also be said about the possible role of the AQVN in this process. We have seen that in a certain way the AQVN defines transportation characteristics of organic molecules in biological systems. Therefore an

TABLE 14

Correlation between spectral characteristics and carcinogenic properties of steroid hormones.

Substance	Wavelength, nm	Carcinogenicity
Oestradiol	225	+
Testosterone	238	+
Mestranol	242	+
Progesterone	240	+
Medroxyprogesterone acetate	240	+
Dimethystrone	240	+
Norethysterone	240	+

AQVN value that allows the approach of an organic agent to a cell component responsible for the expression of oncogenic information is a first condition which must be met by any potential chemical carcinogen. The energy characteristics of an organic molecule might be a second condition required for the expression of its carcinogenic activity.

All phenomena mentioned so far are interrelated, due to links of which we have only a meager understanding at the present time. In our opinion, however, even this is sufficient to point the direction in which we should proceed in order to understand and overcome such a dangerous biological phenomenon as the cancerization of the cell.

We would like to conclude this chapter by mentioning an interesting possibility indicated by the findings presented here. If we hypothesize that oncogenic genetic information describing a malignant cell is a result of evolution, we may logically assume that the DNA of differentiated cells might include, in addition to this information, other data about biological systems which are simpler than the malignant cell itself. If this is true, then the malignant cell must also carry in its DNA, information about its biologically simpler predecessors. This raises the following question: by simulating carcinogenesis might we perhaps unblock this information thereby inducing the transformation of a malignant cell into a simpler form which would be easier to fight. For the time being this represents an interesting possibility, offering some hope that this approach might lead to beneficial therapeutic results.

CHAPTER 6

The Antitumour Activity of Organic Chemical Compounds and their Average Quasi-Valence Numbers

Chemotherapy along with surgical and radiation therapies represents a basic method of treating cancer today. Since in previous chapters we have discussed the correlation between the electron–ion interaction potential — or, in other words, the average quasi-valence number — of organic chemical compounds and their carcinogenic activity, it is natural to speculate how organic chemical compounds which demonstrate antitumour characteristics react.

Figure 11 presents the distribution of 105 alkylating organic chemical compounds which were studied by Golding and Wood of the U.S. National Cancer Institute.[40] The resulting distribution looks quite illogical at first glance. Out of 105 compounds examined 76 belong to the range of potential carcinogens.[41] If we examine the distribution with regard to the number of alkylating cytostatics per 0.1 unit interval of AQVN, then this density inside the area of potential carcinogens (AQVN = 2.4–3.1) is three times larger than outside this area. Eighteen of the 24 alkylating substances, mainly belonging to different nitrogen mustards, producing a 50%-or-higher increase in the life span of systemic leukaemia L1210, have an AQVN of between 2.4 and 3.1.

The unexpected overlap in AQVN values of organic agents which cause cancer with those which cure it leads to the conclusion that "carcinogenic substances have also a paradoxical tumour-inhibitory action...".† Here we will illustrate two possible explanations.

First, we showed earlier that the electron–ion interaction potential (or the AQVN which approximately represents it) is one of the most important physical parameters in determining whether a given organic molecule takes part in a biological process. Accordingly, all substances which in some way become part of the process of carcinogenesis must possess a suitable electron–ion interaction potential (*i.e.* AQVN). Additional more complex physical characteristics of the molecules will then define their precise behaviour in a specific system and determine whether they *initiate* or *inhibit* carcinogenesis, for example.

As for the other possible explanation, we assume that the molecular

---

† See Ref. 24, Sellei *et al*, p. 197.

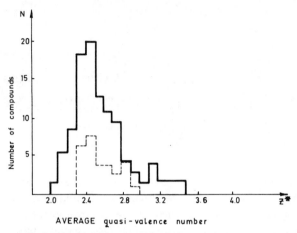

FIGURE 11   Density of the alkylating compounds investigated with respect to their average quasi-valence number (solid line = all investigated compounds; broken line = compounds with good activity).

mechanism of cytostatic action of antitumour alkylating substances is quite diverse and connected with the following processes:

a) the isolation of the structure and matrix functions of the DNA in the process of replication and transcription, during which the reactions of mutation and syndromes of unbalanced growth occur;

b) mixing, in the process of transcription, of the molecules of mRNA, ribosomal RNA, transport RNA, and proteins from the structure of the ribosome. The preceding is the result of the alkylation of DNA;

c) the accumulation of cytostatics in the membrane structure of the cell, which is succeeded by the violation of their function (transmission of electrons and energy, the active transport of substances, etc).

Let us confine ourselves to the interaction of the cytostatics with the DNA, an important process indeed. Suppose that the alkylating cytostatics influence this macromolecule not only when it is in the phase of transcription or replication but also when its information is blocked by the histone wrapping. In this case the alkylating agents must have the chance to obtain the genetic information, that is, to penetrate the inside of the DNA molecule. As we have seen in the preceding chapter, this feature characterizes carcinogenic agents. From this viewpoint, carcinogenic activity which follows antitumour activity of alkylating cytostatics is not paradoxical.

At this point we might ask ourselves why these agents could not influence the genetic information of other sorts of cells in the body. However, *this* question could be asked with reference to the influence of carcinogenic agents:

why do they unblock only the oncogenic information and not information about some other sort of cell which is normally present in the body? It may be assumed that the answers to both of these questions are the same: either this sort of information is not so rigidly controlled, or the physicochemical characteristics of these agents are such that they permit unblocking of only this information, or both of these answers are valid.

On the basis of the conclusions drawn in the preceding chapter, it may be suggested that these thoughts can also be applied to the steroid hormones that are used as cancerostatics. Furthermore if we take into consideration data from Ref. 42, a similar situation seems to apply in the case of cytostatic antibiotics. Later we shall present yet another possibility for which it is unfortunately most difficult to find a fitting argument; despite its speculative nature we feel it is worthy of consideration.

Let us now return to the idea that the genetic information in every cell contains data about our most primitive evolutionary ancestors. This would also be true of malignant cells. Earlier we assumed that such malignant cells result from the unblocking of disfunctional DNA in highly differentiated cells. Thus the possibility exists of unblocking still further genetic information in a malignant cell that would subsequently give rise to the production of a more primitive system than its own. There exist certain experimental facts which support this hypothesis. A certain cell culture, after being treated by carcinogenic agents, maintains the capacity to grow on soft agar. This demonstrates that the higher-level cell obtained, after the influence of carcinogenic agents, exhibits some characteristics of microorganisms. Today this feature of some cell cultures is used as the basis for the most reliable tests on carcinogens *in vitro*.[43]

The other experimental example is no less interesting. A cell culture into whose DNA has been incorporated DNA from oncogenic viruses is treated by carcinogenic agents. In that culture the intensive production of oncogenic viruses occurs, viruses which were only latently present prior to the carcinogenic treatment. Here is another example of unblocking "lower" information in a cell culture under the influence of a chemical carcinogen. As in the preceding case, this method is used for the detection of carcinogens.[44]

In view of this data, we may assume that carcinogenic agents can cause the transformation of a malignant cell system into a more simple one. Such a simple cell system would, according to its characteristics, be more equivalent to primitive micro-organisms which would favourably react to antibiotics. This would imply a therapeutic procedure which would include not only cytostatic but also anticytostatic antibiotics. The contemporary clinical practice of using some anticytostatic antibiotics only serves to confirm the preceding assumption.[24,42] Also, from this viewpoint the simultaneous antitumour and carcinogenic activity of organic agents would be neither paradoxical nor unexpected.

We shall offer a few characteristic examples which will serve to confirm the existence of this bond between the antitumour and carcinogenic activities of organic chemical compounds. For example, urethane (AQVN = 2.77)

has been shown to be carcinogenic in mice, rats and hamsters, following administration by the oral, inhalation, subcutaneous or intraperitoneal routes, producing, among others, lung tumours, lymphomas, hepatomas, melanomas and vascular tumours*.

On the other hand,

this narcotic which was first described by Schmideberg, was found to possess mitosis and growth-inhibitory properties.†
    Hungarian researcher Haranghy applied 1,2,5,6-dibenzanthracene to experimental rat sarcoma and observed good therapeutic results.‡

And further on:

1,2,5,6-dibenzanthracene produced tumours by different routes of administration in mice, rats, guinea pigs, frogs, pigeons and chickens.§

The same is the case with benzopyrene (BP):

BP has produced tumours in all of the nine species for which data are reported following different administrations including oral, skin, and intratracheal routes. It has both a local and a systemic carcinogenic effect.//

On the other hand,

K. H. Brauer's (1963) therapeutic investigations are interesting from both the clinical and historical aspect: he treated human skin cancer successfully with a 0.5 percent solution of benzopyrene in ether.¶

A similar situation exists with methylhydrazine, o,p'-DDD, nitrogen mustard, methotrexate and many other cytostatic antibiotics which are clinically used today. In Table 15 the alkylating cytostatics which are widely used in clinical practice are presented.[45] From these results it is evident that the preceeding conclusions can be completely adapted to them.

    When the other group of antitumour agents, the antimetabolic cytostatics, are considered, however, the situation is quite different. Data for the AQVN of some of them is presented in Table 16. Agents which are clinically in use on a wide scale were chosen. From the results given, it is evident that only one agent

---

* See Ref. 2, Vol. VII, p. 130. † See Ref. 24, p. 194.   ‡ See Ref. 24, p. 197.   § See Ref. 2, Vol. III, p. 187.   // See Ref. 2, Vol. III, p. 115.   ¶ See Ref. 24, p. 197.

TABLE 15
Average quasi-valence numbers (Z^*) of alkylating cytostatics.

Chemical name	Proprietary or other name	Empirical formula	Z^*
1,6-bis(2-Bromoethylamino)-1,6-dideoxy-D-mannitol	Bromodegranol, R-13	$C_{10}H_{22}N_2O_4Br_2$	2.45
Tris(2-chloroethyl)amine	tris-Nitrogen mustard	$C_6H_{12}NCl_3$	2.00
1,6-bis(2-Chloroethylamino)-1,6-dideoxy-D-mannitol	Degranol, R-2, Mannomustine, BCM	$C_{10}H_{22}N_2O_4Cl$	2.45
2-Chloropropyl-biz(2-chloroethyl)amine	Novembichin	$C_7H_{14}NCl_3$	2.00
1,3-bis(2-Chloroethyl)-1-nitrosourea	BCNU	$C_5H_9N_3O_2Cl_2$	2.76
N,N-bis(2-Chloroethyl)-p-aminophenylalanine	L-sarcolysin, Melphalan, PAM	$C_{13}H_{18}N_2Cl_2$	2.54
N,N-bis(2-Chloroethyl)-p-aminophenylbutyric acid	Leukeran, Chloroambucil, Ecloril	$C_{14}H_{19}NO_2Cl_2$	2.47
N,N-bis(2-Chloroethyl)NO-propylenephosphoric acid ester diamide	Endoxan, Cyclophosphamide, B-518 Cytoxan	$C_7H_{15}N_2O_2PCl_2$	2.48
1,6-Dibromo-1,6-dideoxydulcitol	Dibromodulcitol, DBD	$C_6H_{12}O_4Br_2$	2.58
1,6-Dibromo-1,6-dideoxymannitol	Mylebromol, Dibromomannitol	$C_6H_{12}O_4Br_2$	2.58
1,6-Dimethanesulphonyl-D-mannitol	Mannogranol, Mannitomyleran, R-37	$C_8H_{10}O_{18}S_2$	3.20
2,5-bis(Ethyleneimino)-3,6-bis(methoxyethoxy)-1,4-benzoquinone	A-139	$C_{16}H_{22}N_2O_6$	2.87
2,3,5-tris(Ethyleneimino)-1,4-benzoquinone	Trenimon	$C_{12}H_{13}N_3O_2$	2.93
2,5-bis(Ethyleneimino)-3,6-dipropoxy-1,4-benzoquinone	Inproquine	$C_{16}H_{22}N_2O_4$	2.73
2,4,6-tris(Ethyleneimino)-1,3,5-triazine	Triethylene TEM, melamine TEM	$C_9H_{12}N_6$	2.89
1,6-bis(2-Methanesulphonyloxyethylamino)-1,6-dideoxy-D-mannitol	Mesyldegranol, R-49	$C_{12}H_{28}N_2O_{10}S_2$	2.93
1,4-bis(2'-methanesulphonyloxyethylamino)-1,4-dideoxy-meso-erythritol	Erythritol derivative, R-74	$C_{10}H_{24}O_8N_2S_2$	2.91
1,4-bis(Methanesulphonyloxy)butane	Myleran, Busulphan	$C_6H_{14}O_6S_2$	3.07
Methyl-bis(2-chloroethyl)amine	Nitrogen mustard, Embichin	$C_5H_{11}NCl_2$	2.00
6-6Methyl-5-[bis(2-chloroethyl)amino]uracil	Dopan	$C_9H_{13}N_3O_2Cl_2$	2.69
Methyl-bis(2-chloroethyl)amine N-oxide	Nitromin, Mitomen, Nitrogen mustard N-oxide	$C_5H_{11}NOCl_2$	2.20
Triethylenephosphoramide	TEPA	$C_6H_{12}N_3PO$	2.70
Triethylenethiophosphoramide	Thio-TEPA	$C_6H_{12}N_3PS$	2.70
1,2,5,6-Tetramethanesulphonyl-D-mannitol	Tetramesylmannitol, R-52	$C_{10}H_{21}O_{14}S_4$	3.45

TABLE 16
Average quasi-valence numbers (Z^*) of antimetabolic cytostatics.

Chemical name	Proprietary or other name	Empirical formula	Z^*
4-Aminopteroylglutamic acid	Aminopterin	$C_{19}H_{20}N_8O_5$	3.19
4-Amino-N^{10}-methylpteroyl-glutamic acid	Methotrexate	$C_{20}H_{22}N_8O_5$	3.13
8-Azaguanine	8-Azaguanine	$C_4H_4N_6O$	3.73
6-Azauridine	AzUr	$C_8H_{11}N_3O_6$	3.36
2,4-Diaminopyrimidine	Daraprim	$C_4H_6N_4$	3.00
o-Diazoacetyl-L-serine	Azaserine	$C_5H_7N_3O_4$	3.47
6-Diazo-5-oxo-L-norleucine	DON	$C_6H_9N_3O_3$	3.14
5-Fluoro-2-deoxyuridine	5-FUDR	$C_9H_{11}N_2O_5F$	3.14
5-Fluorouracil	5-FU	$C_4H_3N_2O_2F$	3.50
6-Mercaptopurine	Purinethanol	$C_5H_4N_4S$	3.57

(daraprim) is present inside the area of potential carcinogens. Another important fact is that all these agents are grouped above the upper level of the carcinogen area. We shall return to this fact later.

The characteristics of the two remaining groups of antitumour agents, hormones and antibiotics, are, concerning carcinogenesis, completely equivalent to the characteristics of the alkylating cytostatics. Almost all steroid hormones are carcinogenic[†] and in reference to spectral characteristics and AQVN, they satisfy the requirements which correspond to potential carcinogens. A similar situation exists for antibiotic cytostatics (e.g. actinomycins, mitomycin, etc).[‡]

In view of what has been previously stated, we may assume that the physical parameters which are being investigated here can, to a certain extent, help us investigate in more detail the nature of the tie between carcinogens and the antitumour activity of organic chemical compounds.

Let us return to the analysis of the relationship between antimetabolic and alkylating cytostatics. We have observed that the former are situated mainly outside, and the latter inside, the carcinogenic area. If we consider the results for amino acids and purine and pyrimidine bases, we become cognizant of the following: the AQVN range of the alkylating cytostatics completely corresponds to that of the amino acids. On the other hand, the antimetabolic cytostatics overrun the AQVN area of the purine and pyrimidine bases. This observation leads us to the conclusion that the reaction mechanism of these two groups of antitumour agents is different.

This is especially interesting if we keep in mind the data regarding chemical carcinogens which cause neurocarcinoma (Table 8). These also overrun the AQVN range of the purine and pyrimidine bases. In the chemotherapy of

† See Ref. 2, Vol. VI. ‡ See Ref. 2, Vol. X.

TABLE 17

Official National Cancer Institute list of effective antineoplastic drugs and their average quasi-valence numbers (Z^*).

	Z^*		Z^*
Alkylating agents		Hormonal agents	
BCNU	2.76	Adrenal cortical compounds:	
Busulphan	3.07	Cortisone	2.63
Chlorambucil	2.47	Hydrocortisone	2.57
Cyclophosphamide	2.48	Prednisolone	2.63
Dibromomannitol	2.58	Prednisone	2.69
Nitrogen mustard	2.00		
1-Phenylalanine mustard	2.54	Androgens:	
Thio-TEPA	2.70	Fluoxymesterone	2.38
Triethylenemelamine	2.89	Testosterone propionate	2.42
Antibiotics		Oestrogens	
Dactinomycin	2.78	Diethylstilbestrol	2.60
Daunorubicin	3.01	Ethinyloestradiol	2.52
Adriamycin	3.06		
Mithramycin	2.82	Mitiotic inhibitors	
Streptozotocin	3.10	Vincristine	2.76
Bleomycin	3.02	Vinblastine	2.70
Antimetabolites		Miscellaneous	
6-Azauridine triacetate	3.36	Hydroxyurea	3.33
Cytosine arabinoside	3.15	DTIC	3.04
5-Fluoruracil	3.50		
6-Mercaptopurine	3.57		
Methotrexate	3.50		

neurocarcinomas, however, the alkylating cytostatics have an extremely weak therapeutic effect while the antimetabolic cytostatics whose AQVN spread corresponds to that of the agents that cause this specific kind of carcinoma offer much superior results.

For the first time, then, it is possible for us, using a microscopic physical parameter, to focus on the connection between antitumour agents and the basic components of cells. More detailed research into these correlations would certainly help towards gaining important knowledge for comprehending the mechanism of carcinogenesis.

In Table 17 we have presented the official National Cancer Institute (USA) list of effective antineoplastic drugs and their AQVN's (Z^*). In this table we note that different types of medications are arranged around certain AQVN values, with only minor dispersions. Antibiotic cytostatics, for example, are grouped around a value of 2.96, with a deviation of 4.5%; antimetabolics around a value of 3.36, with a deviation of 5.8%; hormones around a value of 2.64, with a deviation of 2%; etc. The only exceptions are the alkylating agents, which are grouped around a value of 2.61, with the largest average dispersion being 11.6%. It is logical to assume that this grouping is not coincidental and

TABLE 18

Cytostatic compounds used in the treatment of acute leukaemias[24] and their average quasi-valence numbers.

Chemical name	Proprietary name	$Z*$
4-Aminopteroyl glutamic acid	Aminopterin	3.07
4-Amino-N^{10}-methyl-pteroylglutamic acid	Methotrexate	3.13
6-Mercaptopurine	Leupurine, Purinethol	3.57
6-Chloropurine	6-CP	3.38
2-Amino-6-mercaptopurine	Thioguanine	3.50
O-d-azoacetyl-1-serine	Azaserine	3.47
6-Diazo-6-oxo-1.-norleucine	DON	3.14
N,N-bis-beta-Chloroethyl-N,O-propylene phosphoric acid diamide ester	Endoxan, Cytoxan	2.48
Vincristine sulphate	Oncovin	2.83
Daunorubicin	Daunomycin, Rubidomycin	3.01

that in some way it is connected with the activity of these agents and to their reaction mechanisms.

In chapter 2 we considered the connection between specific types of cancer and the AQVN values of agents which cause them. We shall now look into the link between certain types of tumours and the AQVN's of antitumour agents which are used in their treatment.

Table 18 lists antitumour agents which are most frequently used in the therapy of acute leukaemia.[24] All of the compounds listed group around an AQVN value of 3.28, with an average dispersion of 6.69%. The only exception is the alkylating agent N,N-bis-beta-chloroethyl-N,O-propylene phosphoric acid diamide ester (Endoxan, Cytoxan), whose AQVN is 2.48.

Cytostatics which are used in the therapeutic treatment of lympho- and reticulo-sarcomas are presented in Table 19. The average AQVN value of these chemical compounds is 2.87, with an average dispersion of 2.37%. Methyl-bis-beta-chloroethylamine (nitrogen mustard) has a greater dispersion from this average value, its AQVN being 2.63.

Table 20 shows the compounds used in the cytostatic treatment of multiple myeloma.[24] These compounds group themselves around an AQVN value of 2.89, with an average dispersion of 2.3%.

A similar situation occurs with other groups of agents used in the treatment of different types of carcinogenic illnesses. It is hardly possible that this kind of grouping, vis-à-vis the AQVN, is purely coincidence; this effect is much more likely to be connected with their activity in malignant cells. Further investigation into this link could prove to be both interesting and important, not only for the preselection of compounds which are tested for their

TABLE 19

Cytostatics used in the treatment of lympho- and reticulo-sarcoma[24] and their average quasi-valence numbers.

Chemical name	Proprietary name	Z*
Methyl-bis-beta-chloroethyl-amine	Nitrogen mustard	2.63
Methyl-bis-beta-chloroethyl-amino oxide	Mitomen, Nitromin	2.80
1,6-bis-beta-Chloroethyl amino-D-mannitol	Degranol, Mannomustin	2.86
1,6-bis-beta-Methanesulpho nyloxyethylamino-1,6-dide-oxy-D-mannitol	R-49	3.00
N,N-bis-beta-Chloroethyl-N'-O-propylene phosphoric acid ester amide	Endoxan, Cytoxan	2.48
p-di-(2-Chloroethyl)amino-d,1-phenylalanine	Sarcolysin	2.86
bis-beta-Chlorethylamino-p-phenylbutyric acid	Leukeran, Chlorambucil	2.79
Vincaleukoblastine	Vinblastine	2.83
Adrenal steroid hormone	Prednisolone	2.91

TABLE 20

Compounds used in the cytostatic treatment of multiple myeloma[24] and their quasi-valence numbers.

Chemical name	Proprietary name	Z*
p-di-(2-Chloroethyl)amino-d,1-phenylalanine	Sarcolysin, Melphalan	2.86
Ethylcarbamate	Urethane	2.77
Adrenal steroid hormone	Prednisolone	2.91

antitumourigenic activity, but also for the advance grouping of active cytostatics which give better therapeutic effects with certain carcinogenic illnesses.

This is extremely important if we keep in mind the intensive process of synthesis and the examination of new antitumourigenic agents. In this field the shortage of rapid and simple methods to determine antitumourigenic compounds presents a special problem. The seriousness of the problem can be grasped if we consider that the National Institute for Cancer (USA) yearly examines up to 50,000 new, and in most cases "absolutely chance," compounds,[46,47] while from the day it was founded until now the medication section of this same institute has examined approximately 250,000 synthetic remedies and about the same number of extracts from natural products.[42] If

TABLE 21

Average quasi-valence numbers and *in vivo* activity of some antitumour drugs.[42]

Name	Formula	Z^*	*In vivo* activity (T/C)† %			
			L1210	P388	B16	LL
(a) Clinical drugs						
Methotrexate	$C_{20}H_{22}O_5N_8$	3.13	272	300	130	N†
Busulphan	$C_6H_{14}O_6S_2$	3.07	N	N	N	N
6-Thioguanine	$C_5H_5SN_5$	3.50	228	132	N	N
6-Mercaptopurine	$C_5H_4SN_4$	3.57	263	150	N	N
Nitrogen mustard	$C_5H_{11}NCl_2$	2.00	160	300	185	N
Dactinomycin	$C_{62}H_{86}O_{16}N_{12}$	2.78	145	275	203	N
Diethylstilbestrol	$C_{18}H_{20}O_2$	2.60	N	N	N	N
Chlorambucil	$C_{14}H_{19}Cl_2O_2N$	2.47	131	198	132	N
Thio-TEPA	$C_6H_{12}SNP_3$	2.70	180	206	N	130
Melphalan	$C_{13}H_{18}Cl_2O_2N_2$	2.54	237	281	257	154
Testosterone propionate	$C_{22}H_{33}O_3$	2.42	N	N	N	N
Cortisone	$C_{21}H_{28}O_5$	2.63	N	N	N	N
Progesterone	$C_{21}H_{30}O_2$	2.38	N	N	H	N
Triethylene melamine	$C_{10}H_{13}N_5$	2.79	168	271	130	N
Prednisolone	$C_{21}H_{28}O_5$	2.63	N	N	N	N
Prednisone	$C_{21}H_{26}O_5$	2.69	N	N	139	N
Hydrocortisone	$C_{21}H_{30}O_5$	2.57	N	N	N	N
Fluoxymesterone	$C_{19}H_{29}FO_3$	2.38	N	N	N	N
Hexamethylmelamine	$C_9H_{18}N_6$	2.55	N	N	–	–
5-Fluorouracil	$C_4H_3FO_2N_2$	3.50	180	220	140	150
Mithramycin	$C_{52}H_{76}O_{24}$	2.82	220	220	N	N
ACTH	$C_{20}H_{24}O_2$	2.52	N	–	–	–
Cyclophosphamide	$C_7H_{15}Cl_2O_2N_2P$	2.48	236	300	167	222
Mitomycin C	$C_{15}H_{18}O_5N_4$	3.05	170	250	167	N
5-FUDR (floxuridine)	$C_9H_{11}FO_5N_2$	3.14	152	255	138	128
Hydroxyurea	$CH_4O_2N_2$	3.33	278	150	N	129
DITC	$C_6H_{10}ON_6$	3.04	150	154	145	N
Vinblastine	$C_{46}H_{58}O_9N_4$	2.70	140	212	220	N
Ara-C (cystosine arabinoside)	$C_9H_{13}O_5N_3$	3.13	2000	221	160	137
Vincristine	$C_{46}H_{56}O_{10}N_4$	2.76	147	242	189	N

Compound	Formula	AQVN				
Nafoxidine hydrochloride	$C_{29}H_{31}O_2N$	2.60	N	–	–	–
Procarbazine	$C_{12}H_{19}ON_3$	2.51	152	160	132	N
CCNU	$C_9H_{16}ClO_2N_2$	2.50	300	272	300	130
Daunorubicin	$C_{27}H_{29}O_{10}N$	3.01	166	267	300	N
Streptozotocin	$C_8H_{15}O_7N_3$	3.15	160	154	N	N
Calusterone	$C_{20}H_7O_3$	2.30	N	N	–	–
Dibromomannitol	$C_6H_{12}Br_2O_4$	2.58	N	170	136	N
Methyl-CCNU	$C_{10}H_{17}ClO_2N_2$	2.50	300	190	234	400
5-Azacytidine	$C_8H_{12}O_5N_4$	3.24	300	253	140	N
1,6-Dibromodulcitol	$C_6H_{12}Br_2O_4$	2.58	152	130	141	N
Isophosphamide	$C_7H_{15}Cl_2O_2N_2P_2$	2.48	215	282	147	154
VM-26	$C_{32}H_{32}O_{13}S$	3.13	300	250	–	–
Adriamycin	$C_{27}H_{29}O_{11}N$	3.06	300	300	300	N
Bleomycin A	$C_{55}H_{83}ClO_{21}S_3N_4$	2.93	N	150	167	158
VP-16	$C_{29}H_{32}O_{13}$	3.05	250	241	280	N
BCNU	$C_5H_9Cl_2N_2O_2$	2.65	300	300	236	172
(b) Some unique compounds						
2,3-Dihydro-1',N-pyrazolo (2,3-a]imidazole	$C_5H_7N_3$	2.80	150	N	141	144
Ellipticine	$C_{17}H_{14}N_2$	2.79	282	204	N	N
a-TGDR	$C_{10}H_{13}O_3N_5$	3.10	158	157	142	N
Fluorodopan	$C_5H_{13}ClFO_2N_3$	2.69	128	168	151	N
Cytambena	$C_{11}H_9BrO_4$	3.12	N	169	N	N
Inosine diglycoaldehyde	$C_{10}H_{10}O_5N_4$	3.45	300	247	186	N
Taxol	$C_{47}H_{51}O_{14}N$	2.90	131	171	N	N
3-Deazauridine	$C_{10}H_{13}O_6N$	3.13	150	N	N	–
ICRF-159	$C_{11}H_{16}O_4N_4$	2.97	166	185	140	130
Dianhydrogalactitol	$C_6H_{10}O_4$	2.90	237	282	166	N
Indicine N-oxide	$C_{15}H_{25}O_6N$	2.68	140	200	153	N
Piperazinedione	$C_{14}H_{22}Cl_2O_2N_4$	2.55	306	214	142	N
Baker's antifol	$C_{23}H_{31}ClO_5SN_6$	2.84	N	N	N	N
5-Methyl-tetrahydroxomofolic acid	$C_{21}H_{27}O_6N_7$	2.98	166	127	132	143
Acridinyl aniside	$C_{21}H_{19}O_3SN_3$	3.02	200	268	278	N
Homoharringtonine	$C_{29}H_{24}O_9N$	2.68	142	300	N	N
Anguidin	$C_{19}H_{26}O_7$	2.77	157	223	N	N
Cyclocytidine	$C_9H_{10}O_4N_3$	3.27	300	224	N	–

Name	Formula	Z^*	In vivo activity (T/C)† %			
			L1210	P388	B16	LL
Nitidine chloride	$C_{21}H_{18}ClO_4N$	2.97	141	238	N	N
Ftorafur	$C_8H_9FO_3N$	3.04	160	134	148	N
1-Alanosine	$C_3H_7O_4N_3$	3.41	182	181	N	–
Maytansine	$C_{34}H_{46}ClO_{10}N_3$	2.74	126	186	145	N
Penta-aza-acenaphthylene nucleoside	$C_{13}H_{16}O_4N_6$	3.13	169	136	N	N
Coralyne sulpho-acetate	$C_{24}H_{25}O_9SN$	3.10	140	190	N	153
Triptdiolide	$C_{20}H_{24}O_7$	2.86	239	150	N	N
AT-125	$C_5H_7ClO_3N_2$	3.11	170	215	127	N
Rubidazone	$C_{36}H_{35}O_{10}N_3$	3.02	180	287	245	N
Bruceantin	$C_{28}H_{34}O_{11}$	2.90	132	217	168	N
Asaley	$C_{23}H_{35}Cl_2O_4N_2$	2.47	158	195	N	N
Di-iodobenzotepa	$C_{11}H_{12}I_2O_2N_3$	2.83	176	232	148	N
Quinolinium	$C_{29}H_{28}Br_2ON_6$	2.76	300	247	N	N
Chlorozotocin	$C_9H_{16}ClO_7N_3$	3.06	300	203	241	N
5-Methoxysterigmatocistin	$C_{19}H_{12}O_7$	3.30	166	206	N	N

† T/C = treated/control × 100.   ‡ N = inactive (less than 125).

we know that this choice of new compounds is not made on the basis of some strictly defined chemical or physicochemical principles but is governed by the use of a structural analogy with agents whose activity is known, then the difficulties of this work are quite apparent.[42] The formation of theoretical criteria based on the use of physical parameters would therefore greatly facilitate the preselection of compounds with cytostatic activity.

The following example will serve to support this view. As a method of screening *in vivo*, the following organic compounds with antitumourigenic activities have been recently used: leukaemia L1210, leukaemia P388, Louis's carcinoma LL, and melanoma B16. Table 21 presents AQVN data and the *in vivo* activities of 80 antitumourigenic agents in wide clinical use today. From this information it is evident that the borderline value of the AQVN which separates compounds which are simultaneously active in more than two test systems from those compounds that are inactive corresponds to 2.70. Considering the 80 compounds presented, in all (with the exception of L-asparaginase, which is an enzyme), 16 compounds are exceptions to this rule (4 compounds which are inactive have AQVN's above 2.70, while 12 active compounds have AQVN's below this level). In any case, the regularity suggested by 80% of the cytostatics in Table 21, deserves our attention in selecting compounds for which antitumourigenic activity is expected.

Of course neither a simple parameter like the AQVN nor the more complex electron–ion interaction potential can, by themselves, constitute a complete criterion. Used in combination with other data, however, such as information concerning structural characteristics, they can considerably quicken and make much more efficient the process of acquiring new antitumourigenic agents.

CHAPTER 7

The Antibiotic Activity of Organic Compounds and their Average Quasi-Valence Numbers

Substances with antibiotic activity form one of the largest groups of chemotherapeutics. Their wide use in the art of healing is apparent. As we have seen, some of them are used as carcinostatics. Here we shall examine the behaviour of these biologically active substances from the standpoint of their AQVN's, since this information will contribute to a better understanding of biological mechanisms which perform in living matter.

In our analysis of antibiotic organic substances with regard to the AQVN (Z^*) relationship we shall make use of data from the recent *Encyclopaedia of Antibiotics*,[48] a volume which covers a great number of antibiotics, giving their molecular formulae, structures, origins, activities, etc. On the basis of molecular formulae known for 1002 antibiotics, we have calculated the corresponding Z^* values and presented the results in Figure 12.[49] In this analysis special attention will be paid to three basic types of antibiotics whose activity on the molecular level is well defined. These are: the inhibitors of protein synthesis, the inhibitors of RNA synthesis, and the inhibitors of DNA synthesis.

Table 22 presents all the inhibitors of the protein synthesis described by Pestka, for which we were able to find corresponding chemical formulae.[50] Figure 13 also presents the distribution of these antibiotics with respect to the AQVN (Z^*). This same table demonstrates, for contrast's sake, the distribution of twenty amino acids with respect to the same parameter. The Z^* was calculated not in reference to the active group but in reference to the total gross formula of the amino acids (Table 6). We can see from this data that of 64 antibiotics which inhibit protein synthesis, 62 fall in the area of Z^* values for amino acids. Only althiomycin ($Z^* = 3.34$) and sparsomycin ($Z^* = 3.30$) do not fall in this area. This is most probably a result of using inadequate formulae. In this regard it should be noted that the molecular weights of those compounds presented in Ref. 50 are not in accordance with the formulae in Ref. 48. Afterwards we discovered that Pestka used for althiomycin ($C_{16}H_{17}N_5O_6S_2$),[51] which is presented in Ref. 52, and for sparsamycin ($C_{13}H_{19}N_3O_5S_2$) from Ref. 53. According to this information, the Z^* values for these antibiotics are 3.35 and 3.04, respectively.

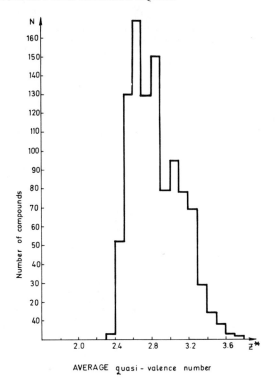

FIGURE 12   Density of antibiotics of all types with respect to their average quasi-valence number Z*.

Let us take a closer look at the correlation of the Z^* between antibiotics which inhibit protein synthesis and amino acids. Table 6 shows the grouping of amino acids around an average value of 2.82, with an average dispersion of 8%. At the same time, the 64 antibiotics listed all group around an average value of 2.78, with an average dispersion of 6.4%. It is evident that both of these groups cover extremely narrow areas of the AQVN with small dispersions grouped around specific average values.

Another important fact is that the difference between the values around which amino acids and protein-synthesis inhibitors group themselves corresponds to only 1.4%. Considering the fact that amino acids are the basic components of proteins and that these antibiotics inhibit the synthesis of these macromolecules, the possibility of coincidence is highly unlikely. Later we shall speculate in more detail on the possible consequences of this fact.

If we examine antibiotics which inhibit DNA synthesis (Table 23), we see that they too group around a value of 3.03 with very little dispersion (5.6%). It is evident that this average value differs from the average AQVN value

TABLE 22

Average quasi-valence numbers of some antibiotics inhibiting protein synthesis.

Name	Formula	Z^*
Acetoxycycloheximide	$C_{17}H_{25}NO_6$	2.73
Althiomycin	$C_{27}H_{28}N_8O_{10}S_3$	3.34
Amicetin	$C_{29}H_{44}N_6O_9$	2.77
Bamicetin	$C_{28}H_{40}N_6O_9$	2.79
Blasticidin S	$C_{17}H_{26}N_8O_5$	2.93
Bluensomycin	$C_{21}H_{39}N_5O_{14}$	2.94
Carbomycin	$C_{40}H_{67}NO_{16}$	2.65
Celesticetin	$C_{24}H_{36}N_2O_9S$	2.81
Chloramphenicol	$C_{11}H_{12}N_2O_5Cl_2$	3.06
Chlortetracycline	$C_{22}H_{23}N_2O_8Cl$	3.04
Clindamycin	$C_{18}H_{34}N_2O_5S$	2.53
Crotocin	$C_{19}H_{24}O_5$	2.71
Cyclohexamide	$C_{15}H_{23}NO_4$	2.60
Dihydrostreptomycin	$C_{21}H_{41}N_7O_{12}$	2.86
Edeine A	$C_{32}H_{58}N_{10}O_{10}$	2.69
Edeine B	$C_{33}H_{60}N_{12}O_{10}$	2.71
Erythromycin	$C_{37}H_{67}NO_{13}$	2.53
Fusidic acid	$C_{31}H_{48}O_6$	2.45
Gentamicin C_1	$C_{21}H_{43}N_5O_7$	2.55
Gougerotin	$C_{16}H_{24}N_7O_8$	3.11
Griseoviridin	$C_{22}H_{27}N_3O_7S$	2.97
Hikizimycin	$C_{13}H_{29}N_3O_{10}$	2.84
Kanamycin	$C_{18}H_{36}N_4O_{11}$	2.94
Kasugamycin	$C_{14}H_{25}N_3O_9$	2.94
Lankamycin	$C_{42}H_{72}O_{16}$	2.58
Leucomycin	$C_{40}H_{67}NO_{14}$	2.59
Lincomycin	$C_{18}H_{34}N_2O_6S$	2.59
Methymycin	$C_{25}H_{43}NO_7$	2.50
Mikamycin A	$C_{31}H_{39}N_3O_9$	2.83
Mikamycin B	$C_{45}H_{54}N_8O_{10}$	2.85
Negamycin	$C_9H_{20}N_4O_4$	2.70
Neomycin B	$C_{23}H_{46}N_6O_{13}$	2.80
Neomycin C	$C_{23}H_{46}N_6O_{13}$	2.80
Niddamycin	$C_{40}H_{65}NO_{14}$	2.62
Oleandomycin	$C_{35}H_{61}NO_{12}$	2.55
Ostreogrycin A	$C_{28}H_{35}N_3O_7$	2.79
Ostreogrycin B	$C_{45}H_{54}N_8O_{11}$	2.88
Pactamycin	$C_{28}H_{38}N_4O_8$	2.79
Paromonomycin	$C_{23}H_{45}N_5O_{14}$	2.83
Pleuromutilin	$C_{22}H_{34}O_5$	2.49
Plicatin	$C_{25}H_{35}N_5O_7$	2.81
Puromycin	$C_{22}H_{29}N_7O_5$	2.89
Siomycin A	$C_{74}H_{92}N_{19}O_{19}S_5$	3.00
Sparsomycin	$C_{31}H_{21}N_3O_6S_2$	3.30(?)
Spectinomycin	$C_{14}H_{24}N_2O_7$	2.81
Spiramycin III	$C_{46}H_{78}N_2O_{15}$	2.57
Staphylomycin M_1	$C_{28}H_{36}N_3O_8$	2.81
Staphylomycin S	$C_{28}H_{36}N_3O_8$	2.81
Streptimidone	$C_{16}H_{23}NO_4$	2.64
Streptogramin A	$C_{24}H_{37}N_3O_7$	2.68
Streptogramin B	$C_{45}H_{54}N_8O_{10}$	2.85

Name	Formula	Z*
Streptomycin	$C_{21}H_{39}N_7O_{12}$	2.91
Streptovitacin A	$C_{15}H_{23}NO_5$	2.68
Tenuazonic acid	$C_9H_{15}NO_3$	2.64
Tetracycline	$C_{22}H_{24}N_2O_8$	3.04
Thiopeptin B	$C_{72}H_{90}N_{18}O_{22}S_6$	3.06
Thiostrepton	$C_{69}H_{80}N_{18}O_{17}S_5$	3.06
Trichodermin	$C_{17}H_{24}O_4$	2.58
Trichothecin	$C_{15}H_{20}O_4$	2.67
Tylosin	$C_{45}H_{77}NO_{17}$	2.60
Vernamycin B	$C_{44}H_{52}N_8O_{10}$	2.88
Verrucarin A	$C_{27}H_{34}O_9$	2.80
Virginiamycin	$C_{28}H_{38}N_3O_7$	2.72
Virginiamycin S	$C_{42}H_{47}N_7O_{10}$	2.92

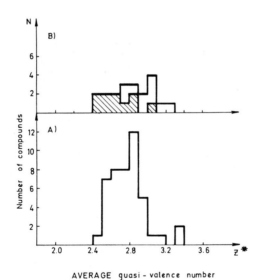

AVERAGE quasi - valence number

FIGURE 13   Density with respect to average quasi-valence number of (a) antibiotics that inhibit protein synthesis; and (b) amino acids (shaded = essential; non-shaded = non-essential amino acids).

around which inhibitors of protein synthesis are grouped. However, it also differs greatly from the average AQVN value of 3.32, around which purine and pyrimidine bases, which form DNA, are grouped with an average dispersion of 4.1 %. The third group of antibiotics (Table 24), however, the group which contains the analogues of adenosine, guanosine, uridine, cytidine and deoxy-thymidine, all of which inhibit the synthesis of nucleic acids, group around an AQVN value of 3.33, with an average dispersion of 6.0%. This value differs by

TABLE 23

Antibiotics inhibiting DNA synthesis and their average quasi-valence numbers.

Name	Formula	Z^*
Antharamycin	$C_{16}H_{17}N_3O_4$	3.00
Bleomycin	$C_{50}H_{72}O_{21}N_{14}S_2$	3.02
Bruneomycin	$C_{25}H_{22}O_8N_4$	3.22
Lucensomycin	$C_{36}H_{53}O_{13}N$	2.72
Mitomycin	$C_{16}H_{19}N_3O_6$	3.05
Myxin	$C_{13}H_{10}O_4N_2$	3.31
Nalidixic acid	$C_{12}H_{12}N_2O_3$	3.03
Novobiocin	$C_{31}H_{36}O_{11}N_2$	2.95
Phleomycin	$C_{53}H_{91}N_{17}O_{32}Cu$	3.00
Pluramycin	$C_{20}H_{25}NO_5$	2.75
Streptonigrin	$C_{25}H_{22}N_4O_8$	3.22
Streptozotocin	$C_8H_{15}O_7N_2$	3.09
Tubericidin	$C_{11}H_{14}N_4O_4$	3.09

TABLE 24

Inhibitors of nucleic acid synthesis and their average quasi-valence numbers.

Name	Formula	Z^*
Analogues of adenosine		
6-Mercaptopurine	$C_5H_4N_4S$	3.57
Tubericidin	$C_{11}H_{14}N_4O_4$	3.09
Xylosyladenine	$C_{10}H_{13}N_5O_5$	3.27
Analogues of guanosine		
Cordycepin	$C_{10}H_{13}N_5O_3$	3.10
Imuran	$C_9H_7N_7O_2S$	3.69
Formycin	$C_{10}H_{11}N_4O_5$	3.37
Analogues of uridine and cytidine		
5-Aminouridine	$C_9H_{13}N_3O_6$	3.23
6-Azauridine	$C_8H_{11}N_3O_6$	3.36
Analogues of deoxythymidine		
5-Azaorotic acid	$C_4H_3N_3O_4$	4.14
Showdomycin	$C_9H_{11}NO_6$	3.26

only 0.6 % from the AQVN value around which purine and pyrimidine bases (and uracil) group, which is 3.35. It is therefore difficult to conclude that this is mere coincidence.

Finally, let us examine, from the standpoint of the AQVN, how inhibitors of RNA synthesis act (Table 25). These substances group around an AQVN value of 2.94, with an average dispersion of 5.8 %. Notable exceptions to this regularity include hadacidin (3.54) and miracil D (2.63). We should keep in

TABLE 25

Antibiotics inhibiting RNA synthesis and their average quasi-valence numbers.

Name	Formula	Z*
Aburamycin	$C_{57}H_{84}O_{25}$	2.80
Actinomycin	$C_{62}H_{86}N_{12}O_{16}$	2.80
alpha-Amanitin	$C_{39}H_{54}N_{10}O_{14}S$	2.97
Aureolic acid	$C_{52}H_{76}O_{24}$	2.82
Chromocyclomycin	$C_{48}H_{62}O_{21}$	2.90
Chromomycin	$C_{21}H_{24}O_9$	2.99
Cordycepin	$C_{10}H_{13}N_5O_3$	3.10
Decoyinine	$C_{11}H_{13}N_5O_4$	3.21
Echinomycin	$C_{50}H_{60}N_{12}O_{12}S_2$	2.97
Gliotoxin	$C_{13}H_{14}N_2O_4S_2$	3.20
Hadacidin	$C_3H_5NO_4$	3.54
Miracil D	$C_{20}H_{24}N_2OS$	2.63
Mithramycin	$C_{52}H_{76}O_{24}$	2.82
Nogalamycin	$C_{38}H_{51}NO_{17}$	2.90
Psicofuranine	$C_{11}H_{15}N_5O_5$	3.17
Rifampicin	$C_{43}H_{58}N_4O_{12}$	2.75
Sibiromycin	$C_{24}H_{31}O_7N_3$	2.83
Streptolydigin	$C_{32}H_{44}N_2O_9$	2.71
Toyocamycin	$C_{12}H_{13}N_5O_4$	3.24
Variamycin	$C_{52}H_{76}O_{24}$	2.82

mind, however, that some antibiotics do not have a completely reliable molecular mechanism of activity.

Taking everything into consideration, the average AQVN value around which certain classes of inhibitors group themselves declines from 3.03 for inhibitors of DNA synthesis, continuing with inhibitors of RNA synthesis (2.94), and finally inhibitors of protein synthesis (2.78). If we consider the location of objects which are influenced by these antibiotics, this decline proceeds from the nucleus to the cytoplasm. It is interesting to note that inhibitors of RNA synthesis group around a Z^* value which is situated exactly in the middle of those around which inhibitors of DNA synthesis and inhibitors of protein synthesis are grouped.

We shall now examine these results from a purely pragmatic standpoint. The problem of the resistance of certain micro-organisms to the influence of antibiotics is common knowledge. The possibility of any antibiotic containing successful activity lessens in time due to the fact that micro-organisms influenced by it at the beginning of its use find a way in time to deactivate it and to both obtain and keep the information about its deactivation in their genes. All of this stresses the need for acquiring even more antibiotics of a natural or synthetic origin to which micro-organisms have no such resistance.

But the task of acquiring new antibiotics is very complicated. A general criterion for restricting the area of organic compounds which might be considered for examination does not exist, as in the case of cytostatics. As a consequence, there is a need to test hundreds of different compounds in order to obtain just one effective antibiotic.

From this standpoint we can speculate how, once found, the correlation between the AQVN and the antibiotic activity of organic compounds might be put into use. As we have observed, each of the three groups of antibiotics analysed covers one specific AQVN area. On this basis it may be assumed that a newly discovered antibiotic will have an AQVN in one of the formerly defined areas, since in the preselection of compounds for testing we mostly start with structural analogues of an established antibiotic. Starting with a familiar carrying structure, different derivatives are synthesized by adding various side groups to it. In this procedure, however, the AQVN of the "base" molecule can vary rather widely, depending upon the characteristics of the adducts. If one or two of the additional groups have a considerable content of hydrogen or halogen elements the AQVN of the final compound can be quite low; conversely, if these groups are rich in oxygen, nitrogen or any other element with a high value of Z^*, the resulting molecule can have a rather high AQVN value. It is clear, then, that a useful criterion for the preselection of molecules to be tested would be to limit the AQVN area to that region where effective derivatives are expected to be found. This approach would help to lessen considerably the number of possible compounds to be synthesized and examined.

The preceding correlation between the AQVN and the antibiotic activity of organic compounds can serve very well as a preliminary criterion for preselection. It would be useful not only from an economic point of view but also from the standpoint of the efficiency of obtaining new antibiotics.

We shall illustrate this important point by using the example of penicillin and its derivatives. The basic carrying structure of this anitbiotic is the bicyclical fragment generally known as 6-amino penicillic acid. It has the following form:

Different forms of the mould *Penicillium* produce various types of this molecule which vary only in the side chain R. For example, one of the penicillins which is widely used, the so-called penicillin G, contains the benzyl group $C_6H_5–CH_2–$ in its side chain and for this reason it is often called benzylpenicillin. The other derivatives of penicillin are shown in Table 26. As we can see, all of these compounds group around an AQVN value of 3.03, with

TABLE 26

Therapeutically important penicilins[58] and their quasi-valence numbers.

Name	Formula	Z^*
Penicillin G	$C_{16}H_{18}N_2O_4S$	3.00
Penicillin V	$C_{16}H_{18}N_2O_5S$	3.05
Penethicillin	$C_{17}H_{20}N_2O_5S$	3.00
Propicillin	$C_{18}H_{22}N_2O_5S$	2.92
Azidocillin	$C_{16}H_{17}N_5O_4S$	3.16
Methicillin	$C_{17}H_{20}N_2O_6S$	3.04
Oxacillin	$C_{19}H_{19}N_3O_5S$	3.11
Cloxacillin	$C_{19}H_{18}ClN_3O_5S$	3.11
Dicloxacillin	$C_{19}H_{17}Cl_2N_3O_5S$	3.11
Flucloxacillin	$C_{19}H_{17}ClFN_3O_5S$	3.11
Ampicillin	$C_{16}H_{19}N_3O_4S$	2.98
Plivampicillin	$C_{22}H_{29}N_3O_6S$	2.85
Talampicillin	$C_{24}H_{23}N_3O_6S$	3.08
Bacampicillin	$C_{21}H_{27}N_3O_7S$	2.95
Hetacillin	$C_{19}H_{23}N_3O_4S$	2.88
Epicillin	$C_{16}H_{21}N_3O_4S$	2.90
Amoxicillin	$C_{16}H_{19}N_3O_5S$	3.02
Furbucillin	$C_{19}H_{24}N_2O_7S$	3.00
Carbenicillin	$C_{17}H_{18}N_2O_6S$	3.13
Carindacillin	$C_{26}H_{26}N_2O_6S$	3.00
Carfecillin	$C_{23}H_{22}N_2O_6S$	3.07
Azlocillin	$C_{20}H_{23}N_5O_6S$	3.09
Piperacillin	$C_{23}H_{27}N_5O_7S$	3.09
Ticarcillin	$C_{15}H_{16}N_2O_6S$	3.27
Sulbenicillin	$C_{16}H_{18}N_2O_7S_2$	3.24
Mecillinam	$C_{15}H_{23}N_3O_3S$	2.71
Pivmecillinam	$C_{21}H_{33}N_3O_5S$	2.67

an average dispersion of only 4%. This means that, in the wide spectrum of possible derivatives of penicillin, special attention should be paid to compounds situated in the narrow AQVN area between 2.90 and 3.10. It is clear that this preselection considerably narrows the possible choice of compounds from the large group of penicillin derivatives to those which could have antibiotic activity.

In keeping with the preceding analysis, we may conclude the following: while searching for compounds which might possess specific antibiotic properties, we can combine knowledge of the active AQVN area with additional information, such as the basic structural characteristics of the sought-after compound, for example, to make a much more efficient choice than can be made employing the approaches currently in use.

Of course, the Z^* criterion is not sufficient in itself, since effects such as structural isomerism, stereoisomerism, dipole characteristics, etc, have a great influence on the activity of organic molecules in biological processes. Nevertheless the correlation we have discovered, between the AQVN of organic molecules and their antibiotic activity, cannot be ignored, especially from the perspective of the design and selection of new antibiotics and with a view toward testing the biological activity of these substances on the molecular level.

CHAPTER 8

The Correlation Between the AQVN of Some Organic Compounds and their Biological Activity

Cytostatics and antibiotics are not the only organic compounds that show a correlation between their AQVN's and biological activities. So far we have demonstrated that the AQVN also plays an important role in vitamins and steroid hormones and we will now show that this correlation is also evident in other groups of organic compounds which have quite different natures and activities.

First we shall look into the relationship between the AQVN of molecules which cause pain and those used to arrest it. One rather familiar molecule which causes pain is bradykinin, a peptide which contains nine amino acids and has the following structure:[54]

$$N_2H-Arg-Pro-Pro-Gly-Phen-Ser-Pro-Phen-Arg-CO_2H.$$

Bradykinin belongs to the group of substances which are secreted at the point of injury, *e.g.* in wounds or in locations infected with bacteria. The introduction of this compound into the bodies of experimental animals also causes bronchospasm, thus causing difficulty in breathing and even suffocation.

Now let us consider substances which lessen pain. Some of them are presented in Table 27. As we can see, these compounds group themselves around an average AQVN value of 2.64, with a dispersion of 4.7%. At the same time, this AQVN value around which the grouping occurs differs from the average value of bradykinin by only 5.0%. It may be assumed that the potential, *i.e.* the AQVN, of these compounds is one of the characteristics which enables them to block the reception of bradykinin and other molecules which inflict pain. At the same time, it is interesting to note that most of these compounds, like bradykinin, cause bronchospasm, which makes their therapeutic use more difficult. Some of them, however, *e.g.* nalorphine, arrest bronchospasm caused by other substances.

Given these facts, we may conclude that the AQVN can play an important role in the preselection of compounds which possess the ability to lessen pain. Most of the compounds in Table 27 are quite similar with regard to their

TABLE 27
Average quasi-valence number of a "molecule of pain", and some pain relievers.

Name	Formula	Z*
Morphine	$C_{17}H_{19}NO_3$	2.75
Codeine	$C_{18}H_{21}NO_3$	2.70
Heroin	$C_{21}H_{23}NO_5$	2.84
Bently	$C_{25}H_{31}NO_4$	2.62
N-Allylnorcodeine	$C_{19}H_{21}NO_3$	2.73
Pentazocine	$C_{19}H_{27}NO$	2.38(?)
Cocaine	$C_{17}H_{21}NO_4$	2.74
Procaine	$C_{13}H_{20}N_2O_2$	2.54
Nalorphine	$C_{20}H_{23}NO_3$	2.68
"Molecule of pain"	$C_{50}H_{83}N_{15}O_{11}$	2.78

TABLE 28
Average quasi-valence numbers of some tranquilizers and depressants.[54]

Name	Formula	Z*
Barbital (Veronal)	$C_8H_{12}N_2O_3$	2.88
Phenobarbital	$C_{12}H_{12}N_2O_3$	3.03
Pentobarbital (Nembutal)	$C_{11}H_{18}N_2O_3$	2.65
Secobarbital (Seconal)	$C_{12}H_{18}N_2O_3$	2.69
Amobarbital (Amital)	$C_{11}H_{18}N_2O_3$	2.65
Thiopental	$C_{11}H_{18}N_2O_2S$	2.65
Pentothal sodium	$C_{11}H_{17}N_2O_2SNa$	2.65
Chlorpromazine	$C_{17}H_{19}ClN_2S$	2.60
Meprobamate	$C_7H_{18}N_2O_4$	2.58
Diazepam	$C_{16}H_{13}ClN_2O$	2.85

structural characteristics, but their AQVN's can vary greatly, depending upon what is added to the basic carrying structure.

This point may be illustrated using the example of the alkaloid group of tropeines. The first member of the tropine order has an AQVN of 2.19, while cocaine, which is practically derived from this structure, has an AQVN of 2.74. The difference between these two values is 28%, six times greater than the dispersion in Table 27.

A similar analysis can be made for the group of substances used to induce sleep, *i.e.* tranquilizers, calming-down substances. Table 28 presents AQVN's for some medications from this group. These compounds group themselves around an average AQVN of 2.74, with a dispersion of 5.5%. Everything previously stated for substances which diminish pain also holds true for these substances. It should be added that the mechanism of activity of these agents has not been completely explained, even today. Researchers in this field are

TABLE 29
Average quasi-valence numbers of some adrenergic and cholinergic drugs.

Name	Formula	Z^*
Adrenergic drugs		
Isoproterenol	$C_{11}H_{17}O_3N$	2.63
Amphetamine	$C_9H_{13}N$	2.35
Methamphetamine	$C_{10}H_{15}N$	2.31
Dopa	$C_9H_{11}O_4N$	3.04
Phenoxybenzamine	$C_{18}H_{23}ON$	2.47
Phentolamine	$C_{17}H_{19}ON_3$	2.70
Ergonovine	$C_{17}H_{23}ON_3$	2.55
LSD	$C_{19}H_{25}ON_3$	2.54
Propranolol	$C_{16}H_{21}O_2N$	2.55
Dichloroisoproterenol	$C_{11}H_{15}Cl_2ON$	2.40
6-Hydroxydopamine	$C_8H_{11}O_3N$	2.87
Cholinergic drugs		
Carbachol	$C_6H_{15}O_2N_2$	2.44
Muscarine	$C_9H_{20}O_2N$	2.28
Acetylcholine	$C_7H_{14}O_2N$	2.46
Nicotine	$C_{10}H_{14}N_2$	2.46
Physostigmine	$C_{15}H_{21}ON_3$	2.55
DFP	$C_6H_{14}FO_3P$	2.48
Atropine	$C_{16}H_{23}O_3N$	2.56
Hexamethonium	$C_8H_{20}N_2$	2.07
d-Tubocurarine	$C_{38}H_{44}O_5N_2$	2.65

especially confused by structurally similar compounds which have a completely different influence on the human body.

Such is the case with chlorpromazine (2.6) and imipramine (2.44); the former
is an efficient tranquilizer, while the latter is a substance which strongly
stimulates the nervous system. In this instance, while from the standpoint of
structure the difference is miniscule, the difference in AQVN values is quite
significant. This is yet another example which demonstrates that in these cases
the potential, *i.e.* the AQVN, can offer important supplementary information.

It is important to discuss the performance of adrenergic and cholinergic
drugs (Table 29), both of which stimulate the nervous system. The latter class
of these stimulants groups around an AQVN of 2.54, with an average
dispersion of 6.6 %, while the former groups around an AQVN of 2.49, with an
average dispersion of 4.4 %. It is thus evident from this information that the
previously found regularity also applies to this group of agents.

Finally, let us offer one more example that bears upon the correlation
between the AQVN and the biological activity of organic compounds;
medications used for curing malaria. According to recent data this ancient
illness endangers approximately one third of the populated area of the
earth today. Approximately two million people die from it each year, while
the number who become ill from chronic malaria is in the hundreds of millions.

TABLE 30

Antimalarial[54] drugs and their quasi-valence numbers.

Name	Formula	Z*
Quinine	$C_{20}H_{24}N_2O_2$	2.62
Pamachin	$C_{19}H_{27}N_3O$	2.48
Atabrine	$C_{23}H_{30}N_3OCl$	2.48
Chloroquine	$C_{18}H_{26}N_3Cl$	2.38
Primaquine	$C_{15}H_{21}N_3O$	2.55
Pentaquine	$C_{18}H_{27}N_3O$	2.45
Chloroguanide	$C_{11}H_{16}N_5Cl$	2.61

The first medication of natural origin used in the treatment of malaria, one which has been in use for over a hundred years, is quinine (AQVN = 2.62). Its chemical structure is responsible for its efficient action. Even in the last century different compounds were synthesized, which are structurally analogous to quinine. Table 30 lists these medications, some of which produce good therapeutic results in the curing of this illness.[54] Compounds from this table group around an AQVN value of 2.53, with an average dispersion of 3.9 %. It may be concluded that together with the structure of these medications their AQVN plays an important role.

This is especially noticeable in the case of chloroguanide (AQVN = 2.61), which has a completely different structure from other antimalarial substances. This indicates the possibility that inside this narrow AQVN area we may find other types of compounds which can be used in the treatment of malaria. Today, when the illness is spreading because of the resistance of micro-organisms to existing medications, synthesis of new antimalarial substances which differ greatly in their properties from those in current use, is necessary. The AQVN criterion may be extremely useful in selecting such drugs.

All these facts demonstrate that the use of the electron–ion interaction potential, *i.e.* the AQVN upon which this interaction directly depends, can substantially raise the efficiency of existing criteria which are used during the preselection and designing of medications from various specialties of medicine. Using this criterion could also contribute to a better understanding of the activity of medications on the molecular level. Furthermore, it could help us to leave behind phenomenological criteria in choosing compounds with appropriate therapeutic characteristics, so that we could move on to more objective and efficient criteria based upon fundamentally natural laws.

Even though drugs are the most interesting group of biologically active organic compounds for mankind, various compounds exist whose biological activity is used in other fields. Until now we have analysed the correlation between different therapeutic characteristics of organic agents and their AQVN's. At this point, however, we shall focus our attention on some of the other biological activities of organic compounds so that the role of the AQVN in such biological processes may be more fully understood.

First, we shall take a look at a group of agents whose specific activity is characteristic. These are substances which certain animals secrete in order to influence the behaviour of other members of their species. They are called pheromones (pherein = transfer, hormon = activate). We will concentrate on those pheromones which facilitate communication between insects.

It has been established through experimentation that various insects react to the presence of extremely small quantities of pheromones (some as small as 10^{-17} mol dm^{-3} concentration). These chemical attractants govern a number of the basic activities of insects: the search for food, the finding of a partner for mating, the choice of a place for laying eggs, etc. The biological mechanism involved in pheromone activity is thought to be extremely complex. Generally speaking the mechanism involves physiological modifications which prepare it for the stimulation which will follow. Also, pheromone "may" and "may-not" tendencies play a certain role in the activity.

The first of these compounds to be isolated was bombical, the sex pheromone of the insect *Bombyx mori*. It structural formula and AQVN are presented in Table 31. The same table gives data for a number of other pheromones, although we will pay special attention to only some compounds in this table.

The female of the rose moth *Pectirophora gossypiella* secretes a pheromone which brings about the sexual excitement of the male of this species. This substance is called propilur. We see from Table 31 that its AQVN is 2.23. While working with only this substance in experimental tests the sexual excitement of the male was not achieved. Subsequent research showed that in order to activate this pheromone the presence of *N,N*-diethyl-*m*-toluamide was necessary. This latter compound, which has a completely different structure from the pheromone propilur, has an identical AQVN of 2.23.

The case of the insect *Anthonomus grandis* is also instructive. The male secretes a mixture of four terpenoid compounds whose data are presented in Table 31. It has been experimentally proved that these four compounds behave like a pheromone in a mixture, while when they are applied in isolation they have no effect. All four have quite similar AQVN values: the first two have a value of 2.21, the second two a value of 2.30. This is reminiscent to a certain extent of the former case of propilur, where both the pheromone and its activator had the same AQVN.

If we consider the AQVN's of the group of pheromones presented in Table 31, we conclude that they, like biologically active compounds analysed earlier, are grouped around a characteristic AQVN value (2.21), with an average dispersion of 4%. This is particularly interesting, given the fact that these compounds differ greatly in molecular size and structure.

D

TABLE 31
Pheromones[54] and their quasi-valence numbers.

Chemical formula	Z^*

2.13

2.22

2.05

2.00

2.23

2.23

2.24

$CH_3(CH_2)_5CH_2O-\overset{\overset{\textstyle O}{\|}}{C}-C_3H_7$
2.23

2.28

2.21

Chemical formula	Z^*
	2.17
	2.25
	2.25
	2.08
	2.40
	2.21
	2.21

Chemical formula	Z^*
	2.30
	2.30

Chemists who study pheromones assume that knowledge about the activity mechanism of these agents might successfully be used in controlling populations of harmful insects. As a result, some of these compounds have already been synthesized. Two such compounds are presented in Table 31. The first, trimedlur, attracts the Mediterranean fruit fly, while the other, heptilbutirat, attracts the moth.[54] We can see from Table 31 that both agents can be classified into the AQVN domain of the other natural pheromones. It might be expected, then, that this criterion, along with the others used in this field, can be used as helpful additional information in the synthesis of new compounds with similar activity. This example of the pheromones provides us with further assurance that the AQVN of organic compounds is connected with various forms of biological activity.

Now we shall turn to what for many must be considered an extremely important characteristic of chemical compounds, toxicity. Considering the importance of this problem, we will spend a considerable amount of time looking into it.

The word toxic covers a wide range of meanings. In its broadest sense it means the capability of a chemical agent to cause the death of a living organism when it comes into contact with that organism. In this sense, then, chemical carcinogens would be considered toxic substances demonstrating a long period of duration and high degree of efficiency. In our analysis, however, we shall consider only that characteristic of chemical agents known as acute toxicity: upon contact with a live organism, substances which possess this characteristic disturb its vital biological functions and cause death in a short period of time.

Even though this dangerous trait exists, man has found ways to put these toxic substances to use. Today, it is impossible, for example, to imagine modern agricultural production without the use of insecticides, herbicides, fungicides, bactericides, etc. These chemical agents efficiently combat all sorts of harmful plants and animals. But in using these compounds a number of problems present themselves. Among these, for example, there is the build up of resistance to the toxic effects of these chemical substances which micro-organisms, plants and animals attain after a period of usage. This gives rise to the need for the development of a great number of new agents.

Hand in hand with this problem, there is of course the problem that some pesticides cause harmful effects to man himself. Recent research has shown, for example, that some compounds from this group are present in the final agricultural products and in that way find their way into man's body. Of all the harmful effects these agents have on the human body, the most important is carcinogenic illness, which, to some extent, has already been experimentally proved.

The development of new methods of testing chemical substances for carcinogenicity together with bigger investments for enlarging experimental capacities around the world have, in the past few years, led to the discovery of dangerous carcinogens among pesticides which are in wide use.[2] In our subsequent analysis of the activity of toxic substances with respect to their AQVN's we will take this into account.

We shall begin with an analysis of insecticides, those toxic substances used for the destruction of harmful insects. These agents belong to different classes of chemical compounds: carbamates, cyanates, esters of phosphoric acid, heterocyclic compounds, etc. Table 32 presents data for 169 insecticides analysed in Refs. 55 and 56. They belong to the classes of chemical compounds already mentioned as well as to some other classes.

Examining these insecticides with respect to the AQVN, we see that of the 169 compounds presented in Table 32 and in Figure 14, 143 (or 84.6%) fall in the AQVN area between 2.50 and 3.20. If we examine the density of compounds in this 2.50–3.20 area with respect to 0.1 unit intervals of the AQVN we find that it is seven times greater than the density, derived in the same way, for compounds in the area between 2.00 and 3.60. Considering the more-or-less even distribution of natural compounds which lie between these limits of the AQVN, this AQVN grouping of insecticides could be interesting from several practical aspects.

First, it is interesting from the standpoint of synthesizing new products. With insecticides, as with some other biologically active substances, we have observed a link between their structural characteristics and their biological activity. But this fact is not enough as a sole basis for selecting, from a group of compounds of similar structural characteristics, those which possess favour-able insecticidal characteristics. Now, however, we may conclude that if

TABLE 32
Insecticides and their quasi-valence numbers.[55,57]

Name	Formula	Z^*	LD_{50}, mg kg^{-1}
Heptachlor	$C_{10}H_5Cl_7$	2.36	90
Alodan	$C_9H_6Cl_8$	2.17	15000
Bromodan	$C_7H_5Cl_6Br$	2.10	12900
Dieldrin	$C_{12}H_8Cl_6O$	2.52	40
Sulphotepp	$C_8H_{20}P_2S_2O_5$	2.81	1
Dimefox	$C_4H_{12}FPN_2O$	2.38	5
Methamidophos	$C_2H_8PNSO_2$	2.93	30
Acephate	$C_4H_{10}PNSO_3$	3.00	945
Phorate	$C_7H_{17}PS_3O_2$	2.67	2
Trithion	$C_{11}H_{16}ClPS_4O_2$	2.91	28
Methyltrithion	$C_9H_{12}ClPS_3O_2$	3.00	180
Ethion	$C_9H_{22}P_2S_4O_4$	2.83	96
Metasystox	$C_6H_{15}PS_2O_3$	2.74	40
Thiometon	$C_6H_{15}PS_2O_2$	2.62	85
Disyston	$C_8H_{19}PS_3O_2$	2.61	12
Vamidothion	$C_8H_{18}PNSO_4$	2.73	64
Gusathion	$C_{10}H_{12}PN_3SO_4$	3.29	10
Imidan	$C_{11}H_{12}PNS_2O_4$	3.29	147
Dialifor	$C_{14}H_{17}ClPNS_2O_4$	3.00	43
Zolone	$C_{12}H_{15}ClPNS_2O_4$	3.06	135
Supracide	$C_6H_{11}PN_2S_3O_4$	3.41	25
Acethion	$C_8H_{17}PS_2O_4$	2.81	1050
Cidial	$C_{11}H_{17}PS_2O_4$	2.97	250
Folimat	$C_5H_{12}PNSO_4$	3.00	50
Medithionat	$C_7H_{16}PNS_2O_3$	2.80	420
Formothion	$C_6H_{12}PNS_2O_4$	3.15	352
Cyanthoat	$C_{10}H_{19}PNSO_4$	2.75	3
Mecarbam	$C_{10}H_{20}PNS_2O_5$	2.87	31
Malathion	$C_{10}H_{19}PS_2O_6$	2.95	1200
Delnav	$C_{12}H_{24}P_2S_4O_6$	2.96	240
Paraoxan	$C_{10}H_{14}PNO_6$	3.13	3
Armin	$C_{10}H_{14}PNO_5$	3.03	1
Methylparathion	$C_8H_{10}PNSO_5$	3.38	15
EPN	$C_{14}H_{14}PNSO_4$	3.14	36
Fenitrothion	$C_9H_{12}PNSO_5$	3.24	500
Dicapthion	$C_8H_9ClPNSO_5$	3.38	420
VC	$C_{10}H_{13}Cl_2PSO_3$	2.80	270
Argitox	$C_{10}H_{12}Cl_3PSO_2$	2.69	38
Bromophos	$C_8H_8Cl_2BrPSO_3$	3.00	3000
Ruelene	$C_{12}H_{19}ClPNO_3$	2.59	1000
Fenthion	$C_{10}H_{15}PS_2O_3$	2.69	250
Phenamiphos	$C_{13}H_{22}PNSO_3$	2.63	13
Tokuthion	$C_{11}H_{15}Cl_2PS_2O_2$	2.73	1134
Merpaphos	$C_{12}H_{19}PS_3O_2$	2.76	227
Abate	$C_{16}H_{20}P_2S_3O_6$	3.15	2000
Cyanox	$C_9H_{10}PNSO_3$	3.20	920
Surecide	$C_{15}H_{14}PNSO_4$	3.00	46
Famphur	$C_{10}H_{16}PNS_2O_5$	3.09	35
Salioxon	$C_8H_9PO_4$	3.18	1
Salithion	$C_8H_9PSO_3$	3.18	100
Dyfonate	$C_{10}H_{15}PS_2O_3$	2.69	8

Name	Formula	Z^*	LD_{50}, mg kg^{-1}
Potasan	$C_{14}H_{17}PSO_5$	3.00	19
Haloxon	$C_{14}H_{14}Cl_3PO_6$	3.00	900
Quintophos	$C_{17}H_{16}PNSO_2$	2.95	150
Dursban	$C_9H_{11}Cl_3BrPNSO_3$	2.90	135
Diazinon	$C_{12}H_{20}PN_2SO_2$	2.66	108
Zinophos	$C_8H_{13}PN_2SO_2$	2.89	5
Quintophos	$C_{12}H_{15}N_2PSO_2$	2.91	70
Pyrazothion	$C_8H_{15}PN_2SO_3$	2.87	36
Maretin	$C_{16}H_{16}PNO_6$	3.15	75
Phoxim	$C_{11}H_{15}PN_2SO_3$	2.97	2500
Trichlorofon	$C_4H_8Cl_3PO_4$	2.80	62
Naled	$C_4H_7Cl_2Br_2PO_4$	2.80	450
Forstenon	$C_8H_{14}Cl_4PO_5$	2.66	7
Gardona	$C_{10}H_9Cl_4PO_4$	2.93	4000
Mevinphos	$C_7H_{13}PO_6$	3.04	4
Ciodrin	$C_{14}H_{19}PO_6$	2.90	140
Dicrotophos	$C_8H_{16}PNO_5$	2.84	22
Monocrotophos	$C_7H_{14}PNO_5$	2.78	20
Phosphamidon	$C_{10}H_{19}ClPNO_5$	2.70	10
Parathion	$C_{10}H_{13}PNSO_5$	3.19	7
Dimetan	$C_{11}H_{17}NO_3$	2.63	150
Pyrolan	$C_{13}H_{15}N_3O_2$	2.85	62
Isolan	$C_{10}H_{17}N_3O_2$	2.63	50
Dimetilan	$C_{10}H_{14}N_4O_3$	2.85	50
Pirimicarb	$C_{11}H_{18}N_4O_2$	2.69	147
Carbaryl	$C_{12}H_{11}NO_2$	2.92	850
Mexacarbate	$C_{12}H_{18}N_2O_2$	2.59	19
Mercaptodimethur	$C_{11}H_{15}NSO_2$	2.73	87
Baycarb	$C_{12}H_{17}NO_2$	2.56	410
Aminocarb	$C_{11}H_{16}N_2O_2$	2.65	30
Propoxur	$C_{11}H_{15}NO_3$	2.73	90
Carbanolate	$C_{10}H_{12}ClNO_2$	2.69	30
Promecarb	$C_{12}H_{16}NO_2$	2.61	74
Mobam	$C_{10}H_9NSO_2$	3.13	234
Allyxycarb	$C_{16}H_{25}NO_2$	2.41	90
Butacarb	$C_{16}H_{22}N_2O_2$	2.57	4000
Carbofuran	$C_{12}H_{15}NO_3$	2.77	8
Formetan	$C_{11}H_{15}N_3O_2$	2.77	20
Meomal	$C_{10}H_{13}NO_2$	2.69	290
Tsumacide	$C_9H_{11}NO_2$	2.78	268
Dioxacarb	$C_{11}H_{13}NO_4$	2.97	107
Macbal	$C_{10}H_{13}NO_2$	2.69	542
Landrin	$C_{11}H_{15}NO_2$	2.62	208
CMPO	$C_8H_8ClNO_2$	2.90	648
Isoprocarb	$C_{11}H_{15}NO_2$	2.62	403
Sapecron	$C_{13}H_{17}NO_4$	2.80	110
Knockbal	$C_{12}H_{17}NO_2$	2.56	470
Bendiocarb	$C_{11}H_{13}NO_4$	2.97	35
Ethiofencarb	$C_{11}H_{15}NO_2$	2.62	411
Aldicarb	$C_7H_{14}N_2O_2$	2.56	1
Tranid	$C_{10}H_{12}ClN_3O_2$	2.86	17
Oxamyl	$C_7H_{13}N_3SO_3$	2.96	5
Thiocarboxime	$C_7H_{11}N_3SO_2$	3.00	5

Name	Formula	Z^*	LD_{50}, mg kg^{-1}
Butoxicarboxime	$C_7H_{14}N_2SO_4$	2.93	458
Thiofanox	$C_9H_{18}N_2SO_2$	2.56	8
Cartap	$C_7H_{15}N_3O_2S_2$	2.83	380
Lethane	$C_9H_{17}NSO_2$	2.53	90
Thanite	$C_{12}H_{19}NO_2$	2.47	1603
Valone	$C_{14}H_{14}O_3$	2.84	2
Penfenate	$C_{10}H_7Cl_5O_2$	2.67	10000
Azinphos-ethyl	$C_{12}H_{16}PN_3S_2O_3$	3.08	18
Azinphos-methyl	$C_{16}H_{12}PN_3S_2O_3$	3.29	17
Bromophos	$C_8H_8Cl_2BrPSO_3$	3.00	4
Bromophos-ethyl	$C_{10}H_{12}Cl_2BrPSO_3$	2.80	270
Carbophenothion	$C_{11}H_{16}ClPS_3O_2$	2.82	30
Chlorfenviphos	$C_{12}H_{14}Cl_3PO_4$	2.76	20
Chlorthion	$C_8H_9ClPNSO_5$	3.38	625
Demeton	$C_8H_{19}PS_2O_3$	2.61	6
Demeton-S-methyl	$C_6H_{15}PS_2O_3$	2.74	40
Demeton-S-methylfon	$C_6H_{15}PS_2O_5$	2.97	38
Demeton-S-methyl sulphoxide	$C_6H_{15}PS_2O_4$	2.86	56
Dialifor	$C_{14}H_{17}ClNS_2O_4$	3.00	50
Diazinon	$C_{12}H_{21}PN_2SO_3$	2.70	150
Dibrom	$C_4H_7Cl_2Br_4PO_4$	2.80	430
Dichlofenthion	$C_{10}H_{13}Cl_2PSO_3$	2.80	270
Dichlorvos	$C_4H_7Cl_2PO_4$	3.00	60
Dicrotophos	$C_8H_{16}PNO_4$	2.84	22
Dimefox	$C_4H_{12}FPN_2O$	2.38	5
Dimethoat	$C_5H_{12}PNS_2O_3$	3.00	400
Dioxathion	$C_{12}H_{26}P_2S_4O_6$	2.88	43
Disulfoton	$C_8H_{19}PS_3O_2$	2.61	12
Endothion	$C_9H_{13}PSO_6$	3.20	30
Ethion	$C_9H_{22}P_2S_4O_4$	2.83	50
Fenchlorphos	$C_8H_8Cl_3PSO_3$	3.00	1250
Fentitrothion	$C_9H_{12}PNSO_5$	3.24	200
Fensulphothion	$C_{11}H_{17}PS_2O_4$	2.91	1
Fenthion	$C_{10}H_{15}PS_2O_3$	2.90	241
Formothion	$C_6H_{12}PNS_2O_4$	3.15	375
Iodophenphos	$C_8H_8Cl_2IPSO_3$	3.00	2100
Malathion	$C_{10}H_{19}PS_2O_6$	2.95	400
Methidathion	$C_6H_{11}PN_2S_3O_4$	3.41	25
Mevinphos	$C_7H_{13}PO_6$	3.04	4
Monocrotophos	$C_7H_{14}PNO_5$	2.93	20
Omethoat	$C_5H_{12}PNSO_4$	3.00	50
Parathion-ethyl	$C_{10}H_{14}PNSO_5$	3.13	6
Parathion-methyl	$C_8H_{10}PNSO_5$	3.38	14
Phenkapton	$C_{11}H_{15}Cl_2PS_3O_2$	2.82	182
Phorate	$C_7H_{17}PS_3O_2$	2.67	3
Phosalone	$C_{12}H_{15}ClPNS_2O_4$	3.06	133
Phosphamidon	$C_{10}H_{19}ClPNO_5$	2.70	16
Phoxim	$C_{12}H_{15}PN_2SO_3$	3.00	2000
Tetrachlorvinfos	$C_{10}H_9Cl_4PO_4$	2.93	4000
Triomphos	$C_{12}H_{19}PN_6O$	2.77	20
Trichloronat	$C_{10}H_{12}Cl_3PSO_2$	2.69	16

Name	Formula	Z^*	LD_{50}, mg kg^{-1}
Trichlorphon	$C_4H_{11}PO_4$	2.80	450
Aldrin	$C_{12}H_8Cl_6$	2.38	40
Chlordan	$C_{10}H_5Cl_6$	2.43	450
DDT	$C_{14}H_9Cl_5$	2.50	150
Endosulphon	$C_9H_6Cl_6SO_3$	2.88	40
Endrin	$C_{10}H_8Cl_6O$	2.40	10
Hexachlorbenzol	C_6Cl_6	2.50	9500
Hexachlorcyclohexan	$C_6H_6Cl_6$	2.00	600
Kelevan	$C_{17}H_{12}Cl_{10}O_4$	2.65	240
Lindane	$C_6H_6Cl_6$	2.00	90
Metoxychlor	$C_{16}H_{15}Cl_3O_2$	2.50	2950
Aldicarb	$C_7H_{14}N_2SO_2$	2.69	1
Isolan	$C_{10}H_{17}N_3O$	2.52	20

favourable structural characteristics were to be combined with AQVN values between 2.50 and 3.20 greater success might be expected in the synthesis of new insecticides.

During our work on the correlation between the electron–ion interaction potential and AQVN on the one hand, and the carcinogenic activity of organic compounds on the other, we wondered if there might be some possibility of connecting these physical values with the carcinogenic *strength* of certain agents. It was difficult arriving at an answer to this question primarily because of problems associated with trying to define a way of measuring the degree of carcinogenicity of an agent. Carcinogenic activity is set off by various factors including specific characteristics of an organism which are difficult to define in only one way.

In the case of acute toxicity, however, the problem is not so difficult. In this case a precise definition of the term "lethal dose" exists. Lethal-dose values for the rat are presented in Table 32 for several insecticides. Taking as a criterion for a very toxic substance the arbitrary lethal dose of 50 mg kg^{-1} we looked to see how the insecticides from Table 32 which meet this condition are divided. The results of this analysis are presented in Figure 15. It is evident that of the 80 substances whose lethal dose is below 50 mg kg^{-1}, 59 fall in the 2.60–3.1 AQVN interval.

Let us remind ourselves that the AQVN interval for all of the toxic substances examined was wider than this, covering the area between 2.50 and 3.20. Furthermore, the distribution of the very toxic agents, based upon an AQVN interval of 0.1, is such that the density of substances between 2.60 and 3.10 is 6.70 times greater than that outside this area. The narrow AQVN distribution of this subgroup of extremely toxic substances indicates that this

D*

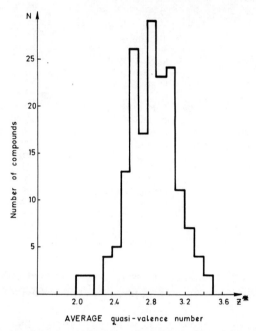

FIGURE 14   Density of the insecticides investigated (Refs. 55 and 56) with respect to their average quasi-valence number Z^*.

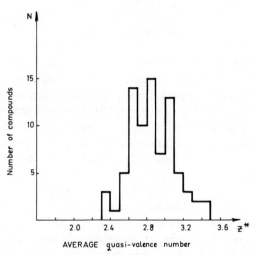

FIGURE 15   Distribution, with respect to average quasi-valence number, of insecticides in which $LD < 50$ mg kg^{-1}.

physical characteristic plays an important role in the functioning of such substances which strongly endanger vital biological processes that occur in living matter.

This correlation between the degree of toxicity and the AQVN becomes even more apparent if we also consider natural toxic substances. These also may be classified using different criteria. According to the most general classification they are divided into two basic groups: high molecular weight toxins (those which are largely protein and protein derivatives) and low molecular weight toxins (generally called poisons). A more specific classification system is based upon the type of chemical structure to which the toxic substance belongs.

It is also possible to classify natural toxins according to the origin of the toxic substance. In this case they would be divided into zoo-toxins (animal poisons) and phytotoxins (plant poisons). This origin method of classification is sometimes more finely made: shellfish poisons, invertebrate poisons, insect poisons, bacterial poisons, mould poisons, rhododendron poisons, etc.

Classification according to the biological activity of toxic compounds is also possible. According to this method substances are divided into stimulative poisons (those which stimulate the cutaneous mucosa) and anaesthetic poisons (those which anaesthetize the nervous system), for example. In our analysis, however, we will use a classification system based upon the organ affected by the toxic substance. With this method we distinguish between cardiac poisons, blood poisons and nerve poisons. We could have used any of the other classification systems, but it has been shown that a simple physical characteristic such as the AQVN cannot follow the specific characteristics upon which those other classifications are based. For this reason we decided to choose randomly toxic substances of natural origin which do not fulfill any special conditions, and we analysed each natural toxic substance in Ref. 57 for which there exists a known chemical formula.

Let us now look at what we might expect to find from an analysis of these substances. Considering the relatively even distribution of compounds in nature, we might expect that at some time in the past there existed organisms which used toxic substances from the AQVN range between 2.00 and 3.00. During the process of evolution, however, those organisms which used the most effective toxins for defense from enemies, or for finding food, had a greater chance of survival. Thus through the process of evolution the most effective toxins should themselves have been selected. Now, if the correlation we have suggested between the AQVN and insecticide activity is correct, and indeed of a more general nature, then we should expect natural toxins which are found in different organisms today to lie in the poison AQVN range between 2.50 and 3.20.

To see how this corresponds to the real situation Table 33 and Figure 16

TABLE 33

Natural toxic compounds[58] and their quasi-valence numbers.

Name	Formula	Z^*	$LD/mg\ kg^{-1}$
Picrotoxinin	$C_{14}H_{15}O_6$	3.06	2
Anisatin	$C_{15}H_{17}O_7$	3.05	1
Neoanisatin	$C_{15}H_{17}O_8$	3.13	1
Phorbol	$C_{19}H_{26}O_6$	2.71	1
Grajanotoxin III	$C_{20}H_{32}O_6$	2.55	0.43
Cicutoxin	$C_{17}H_{22}O_2$	2.49	7
Saxitoxin	$C_{10}H_{19}N_7O_4$	2.95	0.0009
Gonyautoxin II	$C_{10}H_{19}N_7O_5$	3.02	0.009
Gonyautoxin III	$C_{10}H_{19}N_7O_5$	3.02	0.009
Nereistoxin	$C_5H_{11}NS_2$	2.53	–
Cantharidin	$C_{10}H_{14}O_4$	2.79	100
Pederin	$C_{25}H_{34}O_9$	2.76	0.1
Pederone	$C_{25}H_{32}O_8$	2.77	0.1
Tetrodotoxin	$C_{10}H_{18}N_3O_8$	3.10	0.008
Samandarin	$C_{19}H_{30}NO$	2.29	1500
Samandaridin	$C_{20}H_{27}NO_3$	2.55	1500
Butrachotoxin	$C_{27}H_{35}N_2O_6$	2.70	0.003
Bufotoxin	$C_{40}H_{59}N_3O_{10}$	2.63	0.27
Surugatoxin	$C_{25}H_{26}BrN_5O_{12}$	3.25	0.05
Pahutoxin	$C_{20}H_{44}ClNO_4$	2.20	0.176
Aplysiatoxin	$C_{31}H_{48}O_{10}$	2.62	0.3
Debromoaplysatoxin	$C_{32}H_{47}BrO_{10}$	2.62	0.3
Natural insecticides[55]			
Cartiap	$C_7H_{15}N_3O_2S_2$	3.17	–
Nikotin	$C_{10}H_{14}N_2$	2.46	19
Nor-nikotin	$C_9H_{12}N_2$	2.52	–
Anabasin	$C_{10}H_{14}N_2$	2.46	–
Ryanodin	$C_{23}H_{36}NO_9$	2.71	–
Pyrethrin I	$C_{20}H_{28}O_3$	2.50	–
Pyrethrin II	$C_{22}H_{28}O_5$	2.65	–
Cinerin I	$C_{20}H_{28}O_3$	2.50	–
Cinerin II	$C_{21}H_{28}O_5$	2.63	–
Jasmolin I	$C_{21}H_{28}O_3$	2.50	–
Jasmolin II	$C_{21}H_{28}O_5$	2.63	–

present data for the 23 natural toxic substances of plant and animal origin which are described in Ref. 57. From this data we can see that of 22 substances analysed 18 (or 81.8%) are situated in the AQVN area between 2.50 and 3.20. Of these, 13 substances analysed in Table 13 fall in that narrower AQVN area between 2.60 and 3.10 where the most toxic substances are situated. This distribution of natural toxins confirms the general conclusion about the distribution of toxic agents with respect to the AQVN which we came across on the basis of the analysis of insecticides.

This general conclusion is also verified by the distribution of insecticides of natural origin which are described in Ref. 55. Data for these are also given in

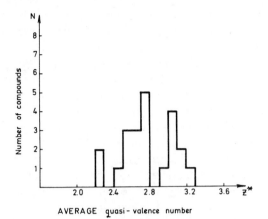

FIGURE 16   Distribution, with respect to average quasi-valence number, of toxic substances of natural origin.

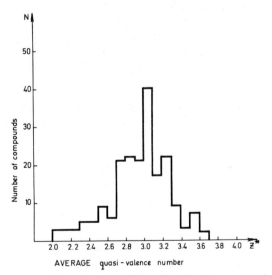

FIGURE 17   Distribution of investigated herbicides (Ref. 55) with respect to their average quasi-valence number Z^*.

Table 33. From 11 of these, only two have an AQVN value outside the area typical for toxic substances. Now we shall check these conclusions on other classes of toxic substances: herbicides, fungicides and bactericides.

We shall begin with herbicides, those substances used against harmful plants. Of 263 compounds analysed,[55] whose distribution is given in Figure 17, 191 fall in the AQVN area between 2.7 and 3.3. If, as before, we examine the distribution from the standpoint of the density of agents using an AQVN unit interval of 0.1, then the situation is as follows: in the Z^* area from 2.0 to 3.9, where mainly herbicides are situated, the density inside the 2.70–3.30 area is six times greater than outside. This means that during the preselection of compounds which would be expected to act as herbicides, special attention should be paid to this area within which lies the greatest possibility of finding active compounds. From an economic standpoint, this kind of selection criterion can be highly significant.

Another important conclusion can be made from the distribution of herbicides. A great number of carcinogenic agents have been found amongst herbicides, insecticides, bcatericides and fungicides, and as a result of advancements in methodology and levels of research more and more carcinogens are being discovered in this group every day. The situation becomes even more frightening when we realize that most of these compounds enter the human body via foodstuffs. Even now no preselective criterion has been discovered that might help to avoid this danger. We believe that the electron–ion interaction potential, the AQVN, offers some hope of being such a criterion.

If we reflect on some of the conclusions drawn in preceding chapters we see that carcinogenic agents mostly lie in the AQVN area between 2.40 and 3.10. Of 263 herbicides analysed, 182 (or 69%) lie in this Z^* region. Almost a third of these compounds are situated in the AQVN area which, according to its carcinogenic potential, is far less dangerous. This means that during the synthesis of new herbicides special attention should be paid to organic compounds from this less dangerous region, thus on the grounds of probability considerably reducing the number of carcinogens among them.

A similar observation applies in the case of fungicides and bactericides. Of 203 compounds analysed,[55] whose distribution is given in Figure 18, 152 (or 75%) lie in the area between 2.70 and 3.40. If we examine the density of these compounds based on an AQVN interval of 0.1, we see that in the area between 2.70 and 3.40 the density of fungicides and bactericides is five times greater than in the area between 2.0 and 3.8. This means that the possibility for antifungal and antibacterial activity of organic compounds is greatest if their AQVN is located in this area.

With regard to carcinogenesis, 124 of 203 analysed compounds fall in the area of potential carcinogens. If, then, we seek a preselection criterion which can accurately foresee the general activity of a substance whilst minimizing its carcinogenic potential, then attention should be paid to the AQVN area between 3.1 and 3.4. This is the only part of the area of maximum density of fungicides and bactericides which is also beyond the area of potential carcinogens.

We shall conclude this section with an inquiry into some possible physical

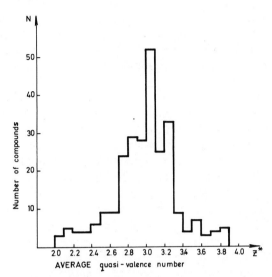

FIGURE 18   Distribution of investigated fungicides and bactericides (Ref. 55) with respect to
their average quasi-valence number Z^*.

explanations for these correlations. It would be impossible to provide completely satisfactory answers to the many questions which might be asked about this problem. Indeed any attempt to do so might lead specialists in areas with which this book deals to question the whole process of relating any simple physical characteristics, such as the electron–ion interaction potential and the AQVN, to complex biological processes about which we know so little. But, as we have demonstrated in this volume, the fact remains that such a correlation does exist between certain physical characteristics of organic molecules and their biological characteristics.

Such correlations were perhaps best described by Wigner:

Between theory and experiment there can exist two sorts of discrepancy: (1) Theory may predict something which is not observed experimentally, and (2) Experimentalists may see regularities for which there is no theory. The first type is relatively harmless (contrary to what some philosophers of science maintain); one can usually find half a dozen reasons why the theory is not precisely applicable to that particular experiment, and one can point to a dozen effects tending in the right direction to decrease the discrepancy. It is the second type of discrepancy which is really serious! If experimentalists find simple regularities for which there is no theoretical explanation whatever, then the theory may well be wrong from the ground up.[58]

But let us return to our efforts to explain the physical background for the correlation we have found. We ask this question: how is it that among the numerous kinds of molecules present the cell unerringly chooses one specific molecule to take part in a certain biological process? It is generally accepted today that structural characteristics of molecules are responsible for this choice. A number of experimental examples leads to this conclusion, in particular the well-known difference in the biological activity of structural and stereoisomers. It is difficult to believe, however, that this is the only criterion used by the biological system to recognise molecules which might become part of a particular process.

Consider, for example, the process of replication of DNA molecules in *E. coli*. During this process approximately 3000 nucleotides come together per second. As a result of errors only one nucleotide in 10^9–10^{10} nucleotides is misplaced. Would this sort of precision and speed be achieved if the recognition of components were accomplished by researching, by the lock-and-key method, the topological characteristics of each and every molecular sort present? It would seem more likely that the system used some much simpler parameter for *preselective* recognition to achieve such great efficiency. Such a preselective parameter might be, for example, the detection of the electromagnetic-field intensity within some distance of a molecule. In this way molecules would be *preselected* which fulfilled a certain criterion involving the strength of the field surrounding them. Molecules needed for a particular function in the biological system would then be singled out by additional selection according to their structural characteristics.

We might inquire as to the origin of the field surrounding a neutral molecule. This might arise as the result of electronic polarization induced by the close proximity of another molecule with a strong dipole moment. Now we know that during such polarization caused by an outer field a regrouping of valence electrons occurs inside an organic molecule. The extent of this regrouping depends on the potential in which the electrons move. But as we saw at the beginning of this book, this potential itself depends upon the electron–ion interaction potential. This means, then, that there exists a direct link between the polarizability of an organic molecule and its electron–ion interaction potential. Having also shown that the electron–ion interaction potential is a function of the AQVN, we may conclude finally that there must be a direct link between this parameter and the polarizability of an organic molecule.

The electron–ion interaction potential can also influence the functioning of some organic molecules in another way. Some chemists hold that the ability of some molecules to react can be seen in the activity of their functional groups which are connected by immovable parts of the molecule. But this viewpoint is only partially correct since collective effects cannot be ignored: a change in any part of a molecule changes the characteristics of all its other components. This means that after the regrouping of valence electrons caused by an outer field the activity of some functional groups can be heightened or lessened. In this way the electron–ion interaction potential can directly influence the reaction capability of molecules.

Having discussed some of the physical causes which lie behind the correlation between the electron–ion interaction potential, *i.e.* the AQVN, and the biological activity of organic molecules, it is hoped that future research in this field will provide more precise answers to the many questions raised. The results presented here demonstrate that this simple physical parameter can be useful if it is built into the existing preselective criteria for all new agents to be used in the environment. The goal is to lessen the number of compounds which require examination, thus leading to a faster and more efficient production of safe compounds which contain the sought-for biological activity.

CHAPTER 9

Conclusion

The results obtained in this presentation may be divided into three basic groups:

a) those related to the preselection of carcinogenic compounds;

b) those related to the mechanisms of chemical carcinogenisis and other biological processes; and

c) those related to the preselection of antitumourigenic agents and other biologically active organic compounds.

In a sense each of these groups constitutes a separate whole. Therefore they will be analysed as such.

Let us begin with the well-known role of the electron–ion interaction potential in the physics of condensed matter. It has been suggested that this parameter may also play an important role in biological processes and, accordingly, in the process of chemical carcinogenesis. This consideration was the initial motivation for our examination which emphasizes the electron–ion interaction potential of a number of organic compounds suspected because of experimental data that indicated carcinogenic activity. With respect to the electron–ion interaction potential and carcinogenic activity, it has been suggested that compounds whose potential lies in the area between 3.30 and 3.80 eV have a greater probability of being carcinogenic than compounds whose physical parameters lie outside that area.

Since in the initial approximation this potential is only a function of the average density of electrons in a molecule, a connection is made between the average valence number and the carcinogenic activity of organic compounds. Results have shown that the largest number of those chemical carcinogens which were analysed lies in the AQVN area between 2.40 and 3.10.

Accordingly, a preselective criterion has been suggested, on the basis of which it is possible, with great probability, to indicate compounds which may possess carcinogenic characteristics. Considering the speed and simplicity with which this criterion can be applied, it is suggested that it will be of considerable benefit in selecting compounds which must undergo lengthy and costly examination.

To supplement this simple physical criterion, the connection between the spectral characteristics of organic compounds and their carcinogenic properties has been used. Experimental results concerning skin cancer induced in experimental animals by u.v. rays prompted this idea, and the results of this analysis have demonstrated that most of the carcinogens examined have an absorption peak in the area between 210 and 260 nm.

Accordingly, we may conclude the following: *organic compounds whose electron–ion interaction potentials lie in the area between 3.30 and 3.80 eV (or whose average quasi-valence numbers lie in the region between 2.4 and 3.1) and which, in their absorption spectra exhibit peaks in the wavelength range between 210 and 260 nm have a much greater probability of being carcinogenic than organic compounds which do not meet these conditions.*

Using this criterion for different groups of biologically active organic substances, we have reached the alarming conclusion that a large number lie in the area of potential carcinogens.

We shall now review the results for antibiotics (Figure 12), cytostatics (Figure 11), neuropharmaceuticals (Table 28), insecticides (Figure 14), herbicides (Figure 17), and fungicides and bactericides (Figure 18). These results were obtained experimentally. Along with the cytostatics, whose cancer-causing properties are already well known, a number of carcinogenic antibiotics are known today such as chloramphenicol, actinomycins, etc.,[2] together with numerous carcinogenic neuropharmaceuticals such as diazepam, oksazepam, phenacetin, phenobarbitone, etc.[2] The problem of pesticides and insecticides is also well known.

From the standpoint of the AQVN, we have analysed groups of compounds from a wide spectrum of biological activities, those collected in Ref. 59. Results of this analysis are presented in Figure 19. Of the 452 compounds which fall in the AQVN area from 2.0 to 3.9, 309 (or 68 %) fall in the area of potential carcinogens between 2.4 and 3.1. This fact becomes even more alarming when we consider that analysis of a few thousand randomly chosen compounds which fall in the potential-carcinogen region of the AQVN values demonstrates an absence of grouping. According to this purely statistical data, which is easily substantiated, we arrive at the following conclusion: the greatest number of carcinogenic agents is to be found among substances which have a function in our bodies. Either we ingest them via foodstuffs or medications, or the body synthesizes them by itself. So it is not surprising that new experiments reveal carcinogenic activity in more and more substances normally produced by the body such as steroid hormones, cholesterol, thiourea and so forth.

We wish to make an interesting speculation in the light of our results, which we feel will be useful in the study of carcinogenesis: these natural substances are not dangerous while they remain in physiological concentrations, *i.e.* in concentrations that can be controlled by the body. If some disturbance or irregularity occurs which causes their hyperproduction, however, then an

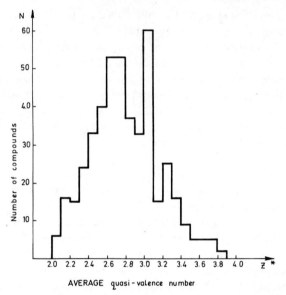

FIGURE 19. Distribution of biologically active compounds (Ref. 59) with respect to their average quasi-valence number Z^*.

unbalancing of the biological processes takes place which the body can no longer control. This same phenomenon occurs, in fact, if the controlling abilities of the body weaken, a fact we know all too well.

Unfortunately, in order to have biological activity many compounds will have AQVN's which lie in the area of potential carcinogens. If there is a demand for a commercial substance to aid a biological function in the body, therefore, and there is no way of avoiding the AQVN area of potential carcinogens, then the compound must be submitted to the most rigorous experimental scrutiny, since there is a significant probability that it will exhibit a carcinogenic activity. During the preselection of commercial compounds designed to have no function inside the human body (e.g. paints, plastics, etc.), we should unconditionally choose those compounds which have an AQVN beyond the area of potential carcinogens.

The second group of results is related to the mechanism of chemical carcinogenesis and other biological processes. Having presented numerous examples in this book, we have demonstrated that a definite correlation exists between the electron–ion interaction potential (i.e. AQVN) of organic molecules and their biological activity. Although we are not able to give a more detailed physical explanation of this correlation, we consider the results presented here to be important enough to warrant the opening of a new area of exploration, one which will certainly not be easy but which will undoubtedly help us to become better acquainted with living matter and its processes.

One basic question which presents itself is how this simple physical characteristic, the AQVN, relates to the complex biological behaviour of organic molecules. At this time it is difficult to speculate whether this is a consequence of its influence on transport characteristics, on the recognition of molecules which are part of some process, or perhaps on something else. Answers to this complex question will be obtained only after a detailed analysis is made of the part played in biological processes by the electron–ion interaction potential.

Some of the data presented in this work, such as the correlation between the AQVN of amino acids and carcinogenic agents, suggest that separation of the energetic parameter as one of the physical and chemical causes of cancer, for example, will be useful in future analyses.

The third group of results is related to physical criteria for the preselection of drugs and other biologically active organic compounds. It has been demonstrated that on the basis of the correlation between the biological activity of organic molecules and their AQVN's it is possible to find an area which will take in the greatest number of compounds expected to possess the sought-for biological activity. Let us hope that this simple criterion, in combination with other currently used criteria, can contribute to a more rapid and more efficient preselection of organic compounds expected to have certain biological characteristics. Surely further exploration into the role of the electron–ion interaction potential in biological processes will contribute to faster and more efficient preselection.

Despite the numerous questions left unanswered, it is hoped that the findings in this presentation will contribute to the opening of a new approach to the exploration of living matter and the processes that occur in it, an approach which will be useful both from the theoretical and practical standpoint.

REFERENCES

1. R. Montesano and L. Tomatis, *Cancer Res.*, **37**, 310 (1977).
2. IARC Monographs: *Evaluation of Carcinogenic Risk*, Vol. I–XVI, Lyon (1972/1978).
2a. IARC Monographs Supplement 1, Lyon (1979).
3. V. Heine and D. Weaire, *Solid State Phys.*, **24** (1970).
4. W. A. Harrison, *Pseudopotentials in the Theory of Metals*, Benjamin, New York (1966).
5. N. W. Ashcroft, *Phys. Lett.*, **23**, 48 (1966).
6. V. Heine and I. Abarenkov, *Philos. Mag.*, **9**, 451 (1964).
7. A. O. E. Animalu and V. Heine, *Philos. Mag.*, **12**, 1249 (1965).
8. A. O. E. Animalu, *Phys. Rev.*, **8**, 3542 (1973).
9. V. Veljković and I. Slavić, *Phys. Rev. Lett.*, **29**, 105 (1972).
10. V. Veljković, *Phys. Lett.*, **45A**, 41 (1973).
11. V. Veljković and D. I. Lalović, *Phys. Rev.*, **B11**, 4242 (1975).
12. V. Veljković, J. Janjić and B. S. Tošić, *J. Materials Sci.*, **13**, 1138 (1978).
13. V. V.eljković, B. S. Tosić and J. Janjić, *Scripta Metal.*, **9**, 459 (1975).
14. B. Veljković and M. Blazon, *J. Materials Sci.*, **14**, 228 (1979).
15. M. Blažon, B. Stanojević and V. Veljković, *Scripta Metal.*, **9**, 1153 (1975).
16. F. Vukajlović, S. Zeković and V. Veljković, *Physica*, **92B**, 66 (1977).
17. M. Davidović, F. Vukajlović, S. Zeković and V. Veljković, *Philos. Mag.*, **36**, 1257 (1977).
18. V. Veljković and D. I. Lalović, *Phys. Lett.*, **45A**, 59 (1973).
19. V. Veljković and D. I. Lalović, *Cancer Biochem. Biophys.*, **1**, 295 (1976).
20. B. T. Matthias, *Progress in Low Temperature Physics*, Vol. 2, Interscience, New York (1957).
21. *Aldrich-Europe Catalog of Organic and Biochemicals*, No. 18, Aldrich-Europe Division, Beerse (1978).
22. *Merck Index*, E. Merck AG, Darmstadt (1961).
23. V. Veljković and D. I. Lalović, *Experientia*, **33**, 1228 (1977).
24. C. Sellei, S. Eckhardt, and L. Németh, *Chemotherapy of Neoplastic Diseases*, Akadémia Kiadé, Budapest (1970).
25. *CIBA Foundation Symposium on Carcinogenesis*, J & A Churchill Ltd, London (1959).
26. J. Arcos, M. Argus, and G. Wolf, *Chemical Induction of Cancer*, Academic Press, New York (1968).
27. C. U. M. Smith, *Molecular Biology*, Faber & Faber, London (1968).
28. A. Szent Gyorgyi, private communication.
29. B. Lewin, *Gene Expression*, Vol. 2, John Wiley & Sons, New York (1974).
30. H. Bush, *Molecular Biology of the Cancer*, Academic Press, New York (1974).
31. B. J. Culliton, *Science*, **177**, 44 (1972).
32. V. Veljković and D. I. Lalović, *Experientia*, **34**, 1342 (1978).
33. H. F. Blum, *Carcinogenesis by Ultraviolet Light*, Princeton University Press (1959).
34. A. I. Scott, *Interpretation of the UV-Spectra of Natural Products*, Pergamon Press, London (1964).
35. M. Terzi, *Genetics and the Animal Cell*, John Wiley & Sons, New York (1974).
36. A. Szent-Gyorgyi, *Bioenergetics*, **4**, 533 (1973).
37. J. Ladik and K. Appel, *J. Chem. Phys.*, **46**, 2470 (1964).
38. C. Heidelberger and G. R. Devonport, *Acta Unio Centra Cancrum*, **17**, 55 (1961).
39. P. Brookes and P. D. Lawley, *Nature*, **202**, 781 (1964).
40. A. Goldin and H. B. Wood, *Ann. N.Y. Acad. Sci.*, **163**, 589 (1969).
41. V. Veljković and V. Ajdačić, *Experientia*, **34**, 639 (1978).
42. H. H. Blohin and C. G. Zubrod, *Sistema Sozdanija Protivoopuholevih Preparatov v CCCP i SSA*, Medicina, Moscow (1977).
43. R. Montesano and L. Tomatis (Editors), *Chemical Carcinogenesis Essays*, IARC, Lyon (1975).
44. R. J. Huebner and G. J. Todaro, *Proc. Natl. Acad. Sci. USA*, **64**, 1087 (1969).

45. L. F. Larionov, *Chimoterapya zlokhacsesztvennikh opukholej*, Akad. Med. CCCP, Moscow (1962).
46. A. Goldin, A. A. Serpick, and N. Mantel, *Cancer Chemother. Rep.*, **50**, 173 (1966).
47. S. A. Scheportz, *Cancer Chemother. Rep.*, **2**, 3 (1971).
48. J. S. Glasby, *Encyclopedia of Antibiotics*, John Wiley & Sons, New York (1976).
49. V. Ajdačić and V. Veljković, *Experientia*, **34**, 633 (1978).
50. S. Pestka, *Molecular Mechanism of Protein Biosynthesis*, p. 467, Academic Press, New York (1977).
51. S. Pestka, private communication.
52. *J. Antibiot.*, **28**, 286 (1975).
53. *J. Am. Chem. Soc.*, **92**, 417 (1970).
54. M. Goodman and F. Morehouse, *Organic Molecules in Action*, Gordon and Breach Sci. Pub., New York (1973).
55. *Pflanzenschutz und Schädlingsbekämpfung*, Ed. by K. H. Büchel, Georg Thieme Verlag, Stuttgart (1977).
56. O. R. Klimmer, *Pfanzenschutz- und Schädlingsbekämpfungsmittel; Abriss einer Toxikologie und Therapie von Vergiftungen*, Hundt-Verlag, Hattingen (1971).
57. *Antibiotics, Vitamins, Hormones*, Ed. by F. Korte and M. Goto, Georg Thieme Verlag, Stuttgart (1977).
58. J. M. Blatt, *Theory of Superconductivity*, Academic Press, New York (1964).
59. *Pharmacopoeia Helvetica* (editio sexta) 1978.
60. H. Gysel, *Tables of Percentage Composition of Organic Compounds*, Birkhäuser Verlag, Basel (1950).
61. A. Efstradiadis and F. C. Kafatos, *Cell*, **10**, 571 (1977).
62. *Bio-Organic Chemistry* (readings from *Scientific American*), W. H. Freeman and Co., San Francisco (1968).
63. C. Kittel, *Introduction to Solid State Physics*, John Wiley & Sons, New York (1956).
64. J. M. Ziman, *Principles of the Theory of Solids*, Cambridge University Press, Cambridge (1972).
65. *Physical Metallurgy*, Ed. by R. W. Cahn, North-Holland Pub. Co., Amsterdam (1967).

Index

A

Acid, amo. *See* Amino acid
Actinomycins, 66, 105
Adrenergic drugs, 85
Adenocarcinoma, 41, 51, 57
Adenosine, 77
Agar, 63
Alkylating agents, 68
Althimycin, 74
Amino acid, 2, 41–46, 51, 67, 74, 107
    chainlike structure of, 50
    role in cell cancerization, 41
    distribution of main components of, 39
    grouping according to AQVN, 50
    hydrophilic type of, 50
    hydrophobic type of, 52
Anaemia. *See* Sickle cell anaemia
Anaesthetic poisons. *See* Poisons, anaesthetic
Animal poisons. *See* Poisons, animal
Animalu, 8
Anthonomus grandis, 79
Antibiotics, 60, 67, 74, 94
    anticytostatic, 63
    cytostatic, 64
Antineoplastic drugs, 67
AQVN. *See* Average quasi-valence number
Arginine, 50, 51
Asparagine, 41
Atomic number. *See* Number, atomic
Average quasi-valence number, 12–107 *passim*

B

Bacterial poisons. *See* Poisons, bacterial
Bactericides 91, 100–101, 105
Bauer, K. H., 64
Benzopyrene, 64
Biochemistry, 3, 47
Biology, molecular, 3, 47
Biophysics, 47
Blocking
    of oncogenic information, 54, 60, 62–63
    of pain inflicting molecules, 83
Blood poisons. *See* Poisons, blood
Bombical, 87
Bombyx mori, 87
BP. *See* Benzopyrene
Bradykinin, 83
Bronchospasm, 83

C

Cancer
    chemical cause of, 1
    of the skin, 64
    preventive protection from, 1
"Cancer DNA", 54, 59
    unblocking of, 54
Cancerostatics, 63
Carbamates, 91
Carcinogenesis
    complexity and solution of, 3–4
    effects of in mammalian systems, 4
    of organic agents, 4
Chemicals
    carcinogenic, 2–107
    newly synthesized, 1
    preselection of, 30
    strength of, 95
Chemistry, quantum, 3
Chemotherapy, 61
Chickens, tumours in, 64
Chloramphenicol, 105
Chloroguanide, 86
Chlorpromazin, 85
Cholesterol, 106
Cholinergic drugs, 85
Cocaine, 84
Compounds, chemical. *See also* Chemical
    compounds
    alkylating, 61
    heterocyclic, 35, 91
    hydrophilic properties of, 47–50
    hydrophobic properties of, 47–50
Condensed matter, theory of, 4, 24, 32, 92, 104
Coulomb, 8, 13, 17
Crystal lattice. *See* Lattice, crystal
Cyanates, 91
Cysteine, 50
Cytidine, 77
Cytoplasm, 79
Cytostatics, 83, 105
    active, 73
    alkylating, 44, 56, 61, 62, 64–67
    antimetabolic, 44, 61–63, 64–67

D

Daraprim, 66
Deactivation, 38

110

Density, of cells, 59
Deoxythymidine, 77
Diazepam, 105
Dibenzanthracene, 1, 2, 5, 64
  carcinogenicity of, 46
Dielectric function, 6–8, 13, 17
  of Hartree, 8
Difractory model, 6
Dipole, 102
  characteristics, 81
  water, 40, 41, 47, 48
DNA, 12, 39, 51, 55, 57–59, 60, 62–63,
    67, 89, 102
  alkylating of, 62
  "cancer". See "Cancer DNA"

E

E. coli, 102
Electromagnetic field
  surrounding molecule, 2, 90, 102
Electron
  bound, 8, 13, 17
  charge of, 8, 11
  cloud density of, 51
  conductive, 6–7, 13
  density of, 51, 104
  free, 13
  gas of, 6
  law of dispersion for, 8
  mass of, 8
  momentum of, on Fermi's sphere, 8
  of closed atomic shells, 7
Electron, valence, 90, 91, 102, 103
Electroneutral complex, 7
Electron–ion interaction potential, 2, 107,
    passim
  method used in determining, 3–7
Electrophilic centres, 51
Embryonic tissue, 54
Encyclopaedia of Antibiotics, 74
Endoxan, 68
Energy, 54, 55, 59, 60
  transmission of, 62
Engineering, genetic, 3
Environment, human, 4
Enzyme, 73
Evolution, 59, 60, 63, 85, 97

F

Fats in human organism, 49
Fermi
  energy of, 26, 32, 33
  momentum, 11
  sphere of, 8

Field, electromagnetic. See Electromagnetic
    field
Food, ingestion of, 36, 87, 95, 100, 106
Formation heat. See Heat, formation
Form-factor, potential, 6–9
Fourier's transform, 13
Frogs, tumours in, 64
Fungicidesm 86–88, 91, 94, 100–101, 105
Furrie component, 7

G

Gastrula stage, 54
Genetics, 3, 4, 47, 54, 59, 60, 62, 63, 79
Glasby. See Encyclopaedia of Antibiotics
Glutamic acid, 41
  in haemoglobin S, 50
Glutamine, 41
Golding, A., 61
Guanosine, 77
Guinea pigs, tumours, in, 64

H

Hadacydin, 78
Haemoglobin, 50
Halogen, 80
Hampsters, 63
Haranghy, 64
Hartree, dielectric function of, 8, 13, 15
Hartree–Fock, functions of, 7
Heat, formation, 12
Heine, 8
Heine–Abarenkov, pseudopotential of, 8, 9
Hepatoma, 41, 63
Heptilbutirat, 90
Herbicides, 91, 94, 99–101, 105
Heterocyclic compounds. See Compounds,
    heterocyclic
Histones, 51, 62
Hormones, 66, 67
  steroid. See Steroid hormones
Hydration
  AQVN as measure of, 48
  process of, 47
Hydrogen, 80
Hydrogen bond, 48
Hystidine, 41